BODY HARMONY

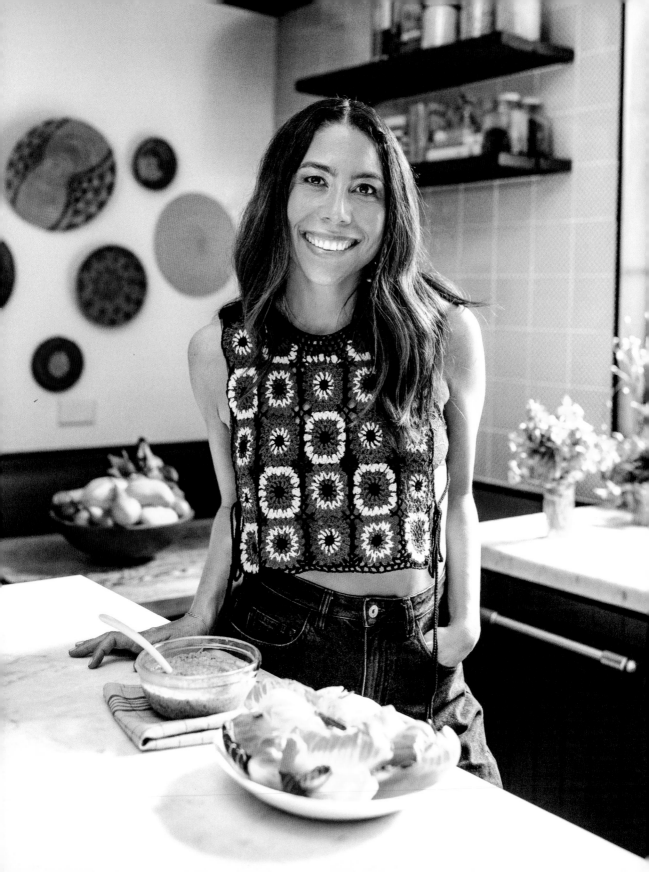

BODY HARMONY

NOURISHING, PLANT-BASED RECIPES for INTUITIVE EATING

NICOLE BERRIE

PHOTOGRAPHS BY SASHA ISRAEL

ABRAMS, NEW YORK

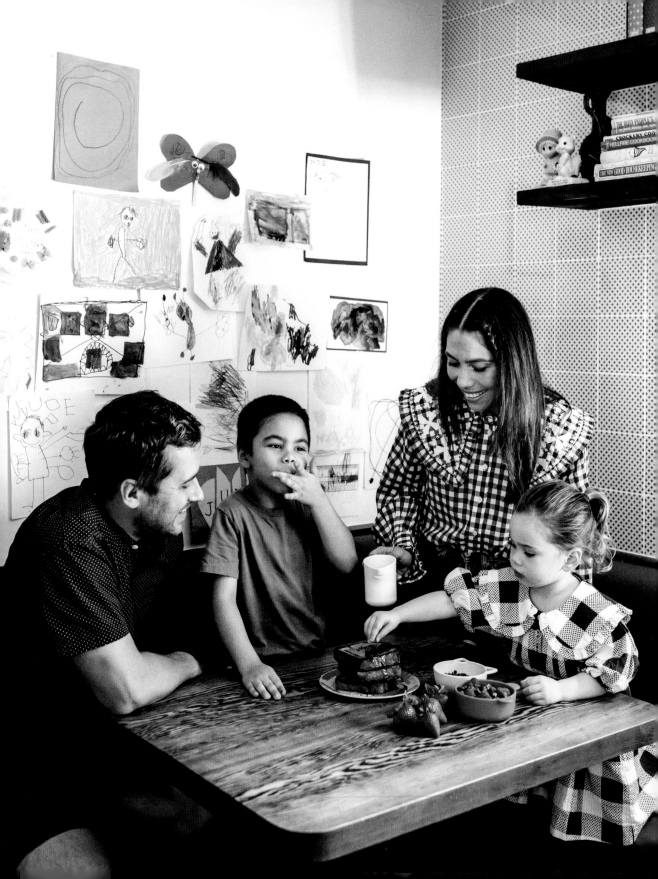

FOR MY CHILDREN, JUDE AND SEA,
FOR MY EVER-SUPPORTIVE PARTNER, NICK,
AND FOR MY DAD, RUSS, WHO HAS BEEN CHEERING ME
ON SINCE DAY ONE IN THIS WORLD AND BEYOND.

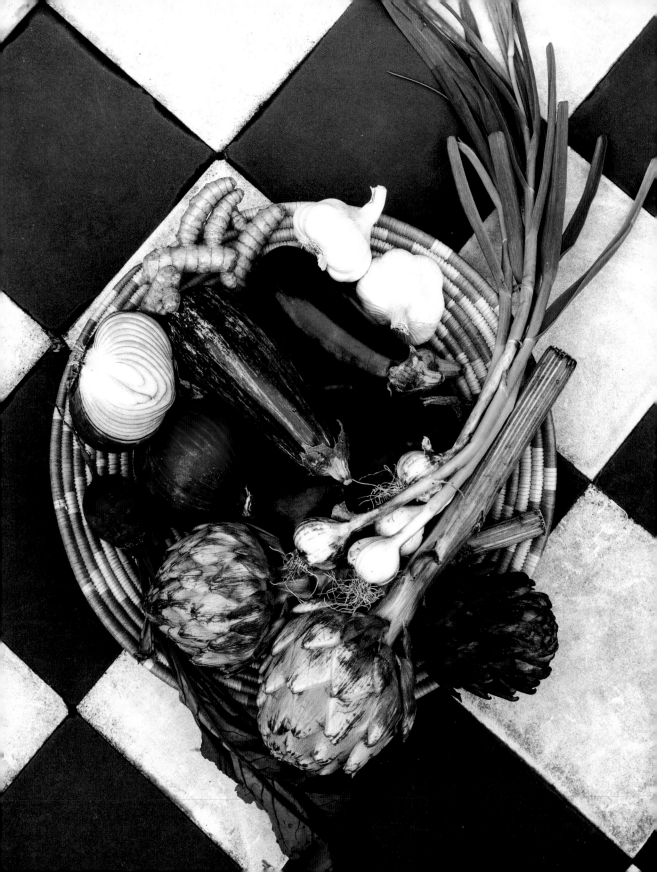

CONTENTS

NEUTRAL VEGETABLES

STARCHY VEGETABLES AND LEGUMES

SOUPS

GRAINS

CONTENTS

IN THE INFINITY OF LIFE WHERE I AM, ALL IS PERFECT, WHOLE AND COMPLETE, AND YET LIFE IS EVER CHANGING. LIFE IS NEVER STUCK OR STATIC OR STALE, FOR EACH MOMENT IS EVER NEW AND FRESH. I REJOICE IN THE KNOWLEDGE THAT I HAVE THE POWER OF MY OWN MIND TO USE IN ANY WAY I CHOOSE. EVERY MOMENT OF LIFE IS A NEW BEGINNING AS WE MOVE FROM THE OLD. THIS MOMENT IS A NEW POINT OF BEGINNING FOR ME RIGHT HERE AND RIGHT NOW. ALL IS WELL IN MY WORLD.

—LOUISE HAY, *You Can Heal Your Life*

Like many people, I have been a seeker of the feel-good. If there was a new fad diet, I was on top of it. I was the overachiever, the perfectionist. Rules felt good. Checklists, to-do lists, and plans outlining my every step kept me safe. But the journey was exhausting. And the destination? Happiness? A glowing vision of health? What was I planning for, really?

Diet after diet, plan after plan, I would follow each outside influence, only to further weaken my intuition at every step. How dare I presume to know what was good for me, when seemingly endless others knew better? The result: I adopted a misconceived notion that, left to my own devices, I was doomed to fail. In my mind, without the discipline of a diet, I would go wild and binge, or forbid myself to eat anything at all. I had numbed myself to my own intuition. Again, like many people, I was taught to distrust that quiet, knowing inner voice that says, "I got you. I'll take care of you. You are safe, you are loved, you are nourished."

It took hitting rock bottom—I'll get to that later—for me to realize I needed a change. That change began simply, with relearning to listen to that quiet voice. And the more I listened, the louder that voice—my own intuition—became. And the more I listened to my body, the better I felt and the more comfortable in my own skin I was.

This book is for anyone who has lost their way around how to nourish their body, having lost trust in their own intuition. In this book I want to help you restore the balance between your body and your spirit, a harmony we were all born with. If you have lost your North Star around food, around the connection between your soul and your body, this book is for you. If you yearn to trust your body and the signals it gives you, this book is for you. If you are looking to cut through the noise of wellness fads and diets, this book is for you. If you long to reclaim peace with your body, this book is for you. If you have already made peace with your body and are looking for more inspiration, for recipes to help get you creative in the kitchen, this book is for you.

I hope this book inspires you to replace diets with approachable, delicious, healing meals and principles that put power back into your own hands. I hope it helps you to rediscover your joy and helps you learn to love to eat again, and to fill your body with abundant, healthful foods. This is the book I needed when I was still searching for answers—a place where I could feel held and gently guided, rather than criticized or forced.

There is tremendous comfort in knowing we can take back power in nourishing ourselves. In the following pages I will explore two philosophies that helped me greatly in my healing journey—intuitive eating and food combining. Intuitive eating is essential, because if we don't first become aware of, and able to tap into, our own intuition about nourishing ourselves, any new way of eating will be just another diet or compulsion. Instead, once we learn to eat intuitively—to trust our bodies first and foremost—then we can use food combining, a method that involves pairing certain types of foods together and consciously not pairing others, as a tool to help our bodies feel the best they can.

The recipes included in this book follow a plant-based philosophy, integrating whole, natural foods into a food-combining framework. They aim to maximize digestion and energy—and raise your vibration energetically. When we eat mostly unfussed foods in a way so as not to interfere with our bodies' natural ability to regenerate and detox, we strengthen our intuition. How? When we feel better, we are naturally guided to more things that make us feel good. When we heal imbalances, like lethargy, brain fog, indigestion, and bloating simply by shifting the way we eat, and when we allow our bodies to thrive naturally and easily, life changes. Miracles happen. Joy happens. Synchronicity happens. This is when the world opens up. We just need to get out of our own way.

I have rediscovered the joy in nourishing myself, which has not only helped me personally thrive but has also become a way for me to show love both to those close to me and to those beyond, through an online community that continues to grow and inspire. Armed with a set of principles that I now instinctively follow daily, I enjoy an unprecedented freedom with all foods. I feel so grateful to be able to share with you all that I have learned on my journey. I hope this book will serve as a guide and a friend in helping you bring harmony back to your body and soul.

With love,
Nicole

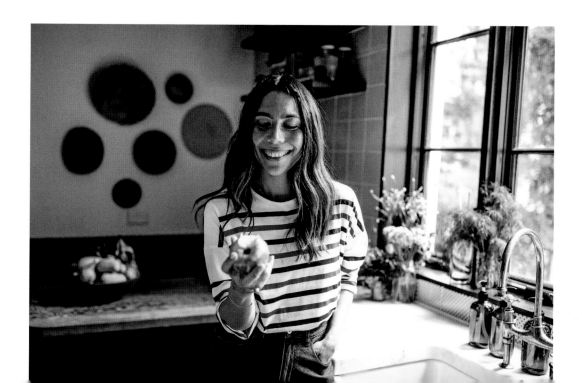

HOW I GOT HERE

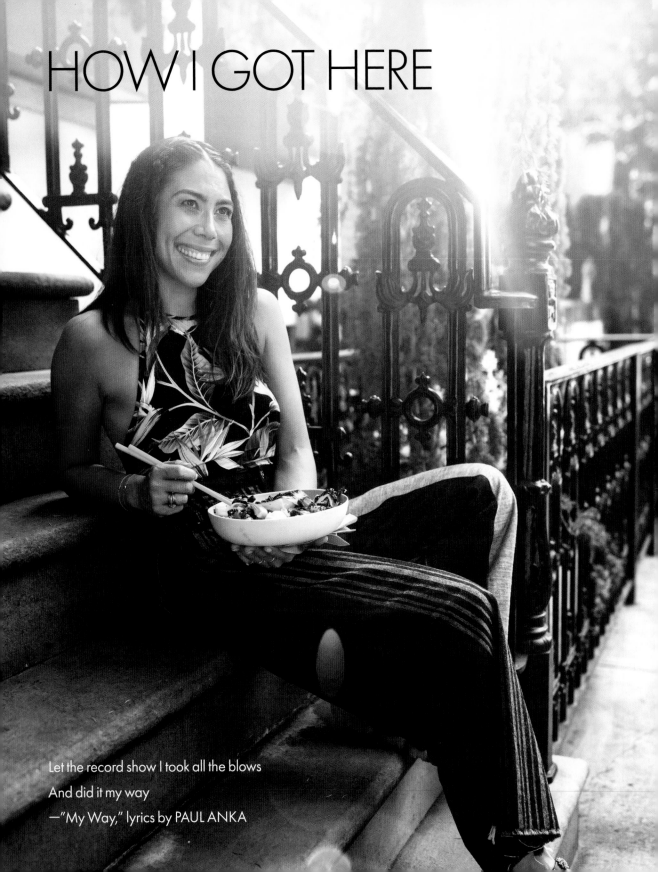

Let the record show I took all the blows
And did it my way
—"My Way," lyrics by PAUL ANKA

A LITTLE BIT ABOUT ME

FOOD AND I GO WAY BACK. Growing up with a father who had type 2 diabetes, I was always aware of how eating directly affected your health. Each morning, I would watch him meticulously measure half a cup of Grape-Nuts cereal and half a cup of skim milk, which he would have with half a grapefruit. This ritual not only comforted me but taught me lessons—positive and negative—about restraint and consistency. There were Sugarless Wednesdays at my preschool filled with "ants on a log" (aka celery sticks with Skippy peanut butter and raisins), seaweed and rice kimbap rolls made lovingly by my Korean grandmother when I visited her in Seoul, and the occasional pastrami and rye jaunt to the Carnegie Deli with Dad. ("I'm being bad," he would grin as he took a big juicy bite of his towering sandwich.) Healthy or not, those were joyful memories. But it wasn't always a picture-perfect relationship with food. Something happened along the way so that I disconnected from that joy and began to fear food.

The Seeds of Fear

My first memory of "detouring away from love and into fear" (a phrase I learned from my mentor, Gabrielle Bernstein) might be when I began carrying a bag of Doritos into bed with me at the age of seven. Each night, I would secretly snack on the hazard-orange cheesy chips while devouring chapter after chapter of *The Baby-Sitters Club*, repressing the guilt that came along with no one knowing my dirty little secret. This was the same time my parents' marriage began to unravel. I would clutch that foil bag like a security blanket as I crunched in the dark while my dad moved his things first into the guest room down the hall, then into a bachelor pad in the city, then into a different house altogether.

Beginning around the same time, I began to suffer verbal and emotional abuse from someone I loved and trusted who used that love and trust as a weapon, exploiting both at their whim and constantly telling me that I was unlovable, crazy, and no good. My heart was stubborn, refusing to believe in my unworthiness, but slowly it began to seep into my soul and I began to detach from my true, joyful self. I was constantly nervous that what I said, what I did, and who I was at my core would trigger the rage of someone I trusted and depended on. When the abuse continued long enough, I began to doubt my innate goodness.

Numbing My Fear

As I grew into my early teens, I tried to bury these painful feelings in alcohol, drugs, and food. I dabbled in the usual teenage suburban extracurricular activities—smoking weed, raiding the parents' liquor cabinet—and this rapidly progressed to going on Ecstasy-fueled benders, dropping tabs of acid at Starbucks, and doing cocaine and ketamine bumps in my high school bathroom. So long as it didn't involve a needle, I was up for it. By age sixteen, I was addicted to cocaine. Simultaneously, I picked up dieting habits from girlfriends and glossy magazines that included drinking shots of balsamic vinegar to speed metabolism, working out in garbage bags to sweat more, and simply not eating at all. This period of deprivation led to a separate period of bingeing and purging, which lasted through college. But I hid it well. From the outside, I was a functioning young woman, but behind closed doors, I was spiraling out of control.

Choosing Food as My Drug

At eighteen, through therapy, I quit using hard drugs but turned to another drug to anesthetize my pain—food. Food had been my first drug of choice. I remember making the discovery, flashing back to those chips on late nights during my parents' divorce—*OH! Food brings me comfort. Food makes me feel good. Food is always there. Food doesn't criticize, hurt, or scare you.* What I didn't realize was that I was using it as a weapon against myself. A clear sign was that no matter what I ate, it was never enough. I was using food to fill a void that it never could, just as I was using alcohol and drugs to escape.

We've all had moments where we have used food outside its first and foremost role of nourishing ourselves. In fact, food had taken on such a bastardized role, I became terrified of it. I was terrified to eat because of the boomerang effect. If it was deemed "good," how long could I keep it up before an inevitable rebound? If it was deemed "bad," how fast could I purge to get it out of me? Nowhere in this cycle was food my friend. It became an enemy. There were times where I would go weeks, months even, without a binge-and-purge cycle, but I felt it looming over me as a dark inevitability. Not once did I go deep enough to examine my feelings, or to examine the hurt girl who was chronically abused emotionally, verbally, and at times physically by someone whom I loved and who I know loved me but was broken themselves. I was a white-knuckled survivor. I kept going. I buried and moved on. Yet my pain and trauma kept me tethered to my past.

The Gift of Grief

I was twenty when my father—my rock, my hero, my best friend—suddenly passed away, from heart failure, in 2002. I had not yet healed from my childhood trauma, so grief was then heaped on top of someone who was already broken. But after a time, grief was the impetus for finally facing my demons. And to feel more connected to my father, I explored a more spiritual path.

It began through reading Thich Nhat Hanh, a gentle Vietnamese Buddhist monk who wrote extensively on anger, presence, and pain. Then I began to read Eckhart Tolle, who spoke of the "pain-body" and stillness. For the first time, I began to sense a presence deeper within. And what a relief that was. I flirted with meditating, bowing, and chanting, but I was still very much planted in the modern world and not quite ready to commit myself to full-time healing.

Bright Lights, Big City

In my mid-twenties, I began an exciting career in glossy magazines where I assisted a photographer who took me under his wing and introduced me to the world of fashion. My life revolved around celebrity-studded photo shoots. It was exhilarating, but my colleagues were searching for the next cleanse or get-thin-quick scheme while peddling body image confidence and feminine empowerment to the masses. We were chain-smoking while downing kombucha. There was a disconnect.

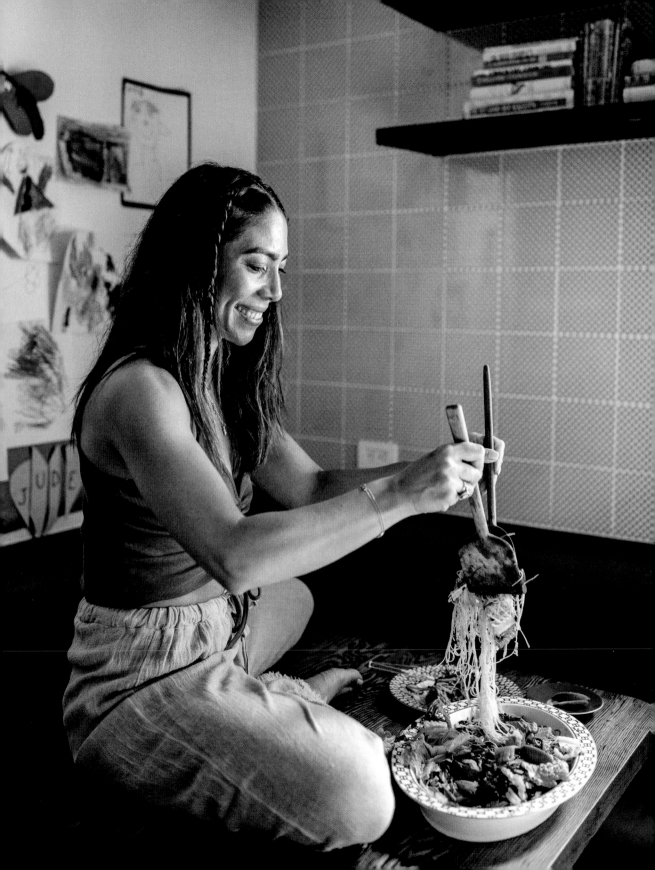

A New Education

One Sunday, I was home reading the *New York Times* Styles section and I came across a cover story describing women in wellness making a career out of healing people. Reading these women's stories lit a fire in me, and I called Gabrielle Bernstein, who was featured in the article as a self-help coach. My phone kept breaking up. Between spotty sentences, "Come over," she said. "I have a feeling we should meet in person." And we did.

We sat on her living room floor. She asked me to close my eyes and we began to meditate. During the session, she called in the terrified little girl who was denied love and tormented for so many years. I began to cry. Silently sob, actually.

She asked me to look at seven-year-old Nicole, to hold her, love her, embrace her, and tell her, *It's going to be okay. She is taken care of now. She is loved. She is not responsible. It's not her fault.* With tears streaming down my face, I felt decades-old walls crumbling. I felt the weight that I carried like a badge of false pride on my heart fall. I felt exhausted. I felt relieved.

This marked the beginning of my healing journey. I made it my full-time job to care for myself, which I realize is a great privilege, and I do not take that lightly. But my life needed to come to a full stop to be able to start again. I began to attend lectures, workshops, anything that felt reparative to my soul. The workshops were the most healing for me. We were a small group of women, equally suffering. Equally carrying stories of trauma and pain and equally determined to heal together. We cried, we journaled, we chanted, we prayed. We stayed late after our meetings and would go for macrobiotic meals. I began to form friendships outside the fast-paced fashion world, the nightlife world. I began to

have meaningful relationships. Real conversations. Real support. I will never forget the women who held me during this time. We would attend lectures, armed with our blank notebooks and pens, and we would scribble notes down while tears silently streamed from our eyes. Then we would go for dinner and talk about *The Real Housewives* over fermented miso soup and yuba rolls.

Here, Now

As I delved more into learning about spirituality, health, and well-being, I quit my job and took a leap of faith to heal myself.

It was during my healing journey that I felt compelled to share my learning, and in 2013, I launched bonberi.com with my friend Vanessa. Our tagline was "A curated guide to well-being." We featured people in all walks of life, from artists and chefs to designers and models, but instead of focusing on their wardrobe or music choices, we asked them about their healing practices: How did they approach nourishing themselves, and what wellness nonnegotiables did they follow? The website was a way to connect my publishing experience with my passion for holistic living. As we gained a following, the focus began to shift to the recipes I developed for the site, and in 2015, right after I had my son, Jude, I decided to relaunch it on my own as a plant-based recipe site featuring not only my dishes but also tips on the food-combining lifestyle.

In September 2018, I opened Bonberi Mart in New York City, a plant-based convenience store that sold my salads, grain bowls, and dressings and a curated mix of healthy snacks, clean beauty products, and nontoxic home offerings. It was not only a destination for people to try all the recipes I had shared over the years but also a place to commune, learn, and heal. In the beginning, we would hold Wellness Wednesdays on which we hosted panels with women in food; we did Full Moon workshops and plant-based facials. Some days, I would sit at the coffee bar of our first location, answering emails, and I'd overhear girlfriends who'd met over salad to discuss breakups, makeups, and reawakenings, not afraid to get deep, cry, and heal in the light of day.

I think back to that article I read so many years ago, about the handful of women who had made a career from sharing their passion to heal. I recognize how my heart ached to do the same. Have you ever felt that? An aching that occurs when you see people achieving all their desires and living out their true purpose. Sometimes we might feel a tinge of jealousy or judgment, but if we look beyond that, we can see we have simply identified the life our heart intuitively wants to live. I can honestly say that the minute I began to live, eat, work, and operate intuitively was when I began the journey to the life of my dreams. But I could not follow my intuition and go for it if I was constantly listening to outside influences telling me what to do with my life, let alone what to eat and when. It was when I started to make my voice the loudest, and I mean that deep guttural voice that is free of judgment and criticism, that my life truly began to change.

Today, bonberi.com and Bonberi Mart continue to grow and continue to be resources for many who have set out on their own healing journeys. I am incredibly proud of how many people have been touched and fed and helped to heal over the years. As a mother, I feel more expansive than ever and grounded in my dedication to lead a healed, fulfilled life, not only for myself but also my children, my husband, and the people in my life. And my gratitude for that continues to heal me every day.

Going Through the Fire

If you are reading this book and you've experienced any type of pain or hardship but are the so-called strong girl, the one who can overthink it, oversnark it, and rise above it: I've been there. I know what that's like, and I know that it hurts. But the only way out of the fire is through it. It's scary, it can be painful, but, holy shit, is it worth it.

Perhaps the greatest miracle is that I have found the courage to heal myself. But it's important to note that my healing is never complete. It's an ongoing journey with ebbs and flows, challenging times, and really fucking challenging times, but I have the tools to recalibrate and reground whenever I feel off balance. I have the wherewithal to be open to new modalities of healing when old routines no longer serve me. That is the beauty of following your intuition. It is always changing and growing, therefore when we follow our intuition, we are always changing and growing. It's also an imperfect path that will look messy at times. Remember, going for your dreams and achieving harmony in your body and your life can mean doing it all imperfectly and making mistakes. (Perfectionists, I'm talking to you.) It means messing up, acknowledging it, and learning from your mistakes. And that is the beauty of healing. In this book, I share an arsenal of nourishing recipes and the tools to help you discover and rediscover what ignites joy in your body and spirit and to truly live a harmonious life.

Are you ready to get started?

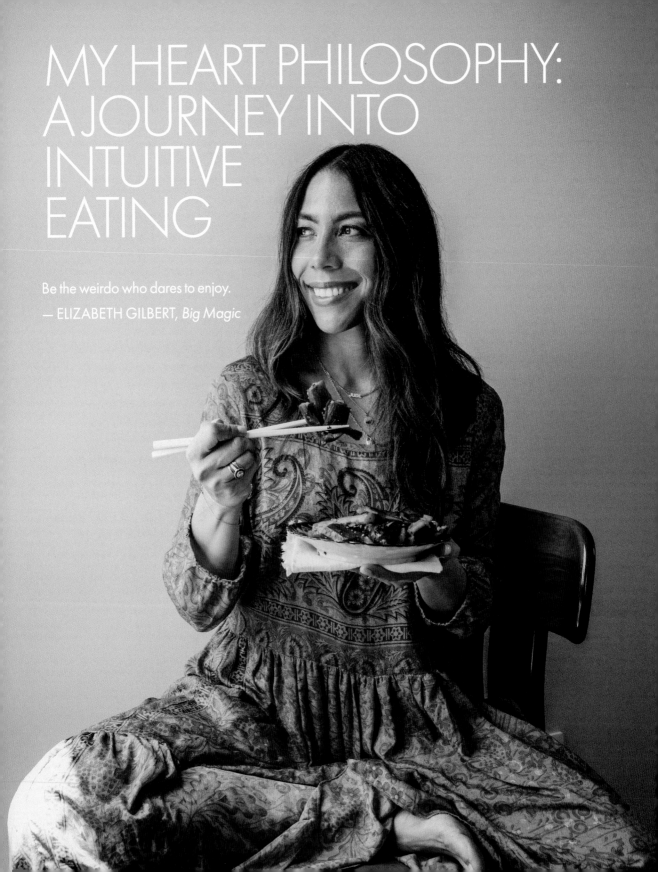

MY HEART PHILOSOPHY: A JOURNEY INTO INTUITIVE EATING

Be the weirdo who dares to enjoy.
— ELIZABETH GILBERT, *Big Magic*

OUR BODIES ARE DIVINELY INTELLIGENT AND WILL ALWAYS SEEK TRUE NOURISHMENT. READ THAT AGAIN.

We were all born with the innate knowledge of how to thrive. But that small guiding voice that was once clear, in our childhood, has gotten lost in the noise of diet fads and #fitspo tags. Remember when you were a child, and food simply equaled joy? It could be the grilled cheese Dad made you after school. It could be the fruit salad Mom would whip up when friends came over. Whatever it was, food was simply a means of nourishment, love, and joy. How do we get back to that child's easy relationship with food? Intuitive eating.

As someone who has struggled with eating disorders—binge eating, emotional eating—and disconnection from my body, I understand what an overwhelming and sometimes impossible feat it can be to reconcile yourself with food. This chapter seeks to set you on the path toward freedom, one small step at a time. And if you don't feel disconnected from your body, bravo, you! Think of this chapter, then, as a gentle affirmation or reminder to always choose your intuition first, no matter what noise is around you.

How the Wellness Industry Has Confused Us

We live in a world of Wellness 2.0, surrounded by many empowering, yet often conflicting messages: Drink celery juice! Whatever you do, don't drink celery juice! Fruit is the best thing for you! OMG, don't so much as look at fruit! These days, we are assaulted by well-meaning armies of nutritionists, coaches, and "experts" telling us what to do. There are brands popping up each day touting the new magic bullet or fountain of youth. Get-thin-quick schemes have given way to get-"vibey"-quick schemes. One camp denounces the other and we're left confused and feeling lost. It's no wonder the notion of healing ourselves can seem insurmountable and entirely intimidating.

Commercially processed and chemical-laden foods and products in our homes have left us tired, stressed, and sick. So in some ways, the turn to wellness is an amazing thing. The fact that the public consciousness is shifting to nontoxic, healthy, sustainable ways of life is incredibly positive. The issue is there are so many points of view, it's difficult to know what's right for you. So you're left feeling helpless. Intuitive eating helps you tune out those outside voices and tune into your inner voice, the one that naturally knows what's best for you.

After years and years of listening to everyone but ourselves, we are desperate to find ourselves and remember how to feel good. I say "remember," not "learn," because—I repeat—we were all born with the innate knowledge of how to thrive. It's the outside world that has made us believe we need a prescriptive plan in order to properly function. But what if someone told us, "You know best"? How would that feel? Probably scary, at first. But once you begin to test the waters of following your intuition, you'll never want to give up that liberation.

What Is Wellness, Really?

Let's simplify things. Wellness, to me, lies simply in the word *well*: How can we feel well? This might mean something very different to me than it means to you. And that, my friend, is the point. There is no one size fits all when it comes to well-being. We are beautiful, wildly unique, ever-changing sentient beings. In fact, what wellness meant to me in my twenties is entirely different from what it means to me now in my late thirties. What nourishes me in January is something entirely different from what nourishes me in July. This is why listening to our intuition creates grace, balance, and flow—our needs fluctuate. What remains constant is the ability to tap in and listen to what our body is craving in that moment.

Get Honest

First, we must get honest with ourselves and acknowledge that any recovery process is a journey.

A journey with highs and lows, detours and pivots. Success is not linear. Healing is not linear. Sometimes, things will get worse before they get better because we are finally shining a light on painful trauma, however big or small, that we have not dealt with for years. But we must honor our old wounds in order to free ourselves from self-destructive patterns.

When we take an honest inventory of our life, we must remember throughout this process to treat ourselves as our own patient. As my favorite writer, Nora Ephron, remarked, "Insane people are always sure that they are fine. It is only the sane people who are willing to admit that they are crazy." She was joking, but the truth is, it is the sanest thing to be honest with yourself.

Have Patience

Imagine yourself as a little girl or boy, an innocent child who does not know any better. Would we scold that little child for not getting something correct right away? Would we punish or judge him or her for trying but then making a mistake? Of course not. We would give her comfort and love and say, that's okay, sweetie, you tried your best and we'll keep going. There may be moments where certain places, meals, or people trigger us into repeating old vicious cycles. That is simply a sign that there is something that remains to be healed. I have used the steps that follow in my own recovery and found that, after consistent application, I was able to overcome my destructive relationship with food and reignite the love of myself, my body, and nourishing foods.

THE STEPS TO HEALING

Get Quiet

"Our breathing is the link between our body and our mind. Sometimes our mind is thinking of one thing and our body is doing another, and mind and body are not unified," writes Thich Nhat Hanh in *Peace Is Every Step*. "By concentrating on our breathing, 'In' and 'Out,' we are bringing body and mind back together and become whole again. Conscious breathing is an important bridge."

Don't be surprised if, when you begin to allow yourself to feel, it might feel like too much. For me, the first hurdle was facing all the feelings and pain I had been trying to numb over the years with food, alcohol, and drugs. It wasn't until I faced those feelings and felt them through meditation, journaling, and much self-work that I was able to release myself from them.

Just breathe and take one moment at a time, asking the universe to support you. You may cry. I did, for what seemed like forever. At first, they were tears of pain, but they soon turned into tears of joy and gratitude that I was finally letting in and letting go. An interesting thing happened. As I shed tears, I began to also shed physical weight that I had been carrying with me for years and that also began to no longer serve me. This weight had a purpose—to protect me from looking at my truth and the pain I was carrying. This is not a weight loss book, but as we shine a light onto our wounds, there is no more shrinking in the darkness or hiding behind our pain, and sometimes we will shed the things that are no longer serving us, whether that be a toxic relationship, a job we no longer connect with, or weight we no longer need to carry. We can expand our energy in the light and truly shape-shift into a new being.

Say No

For most of my early life, I was a classic yes-(wo)man, a people pleaser extraordinaire who was always wondering how I could erase or bend myself enough to accommodate others' feelings and, hopefully, get them to like or love me. This all changed when I made the conscious decision to put myself first, which meant learning to say no—almost all the time.

> The wound is the place where Light enters you.
>
> —RUMI

Saying no is groundbreaking, especially if you haven't done it before. It takes courage to say no, but once you start, it's hard to go back. I don't mean saying no to hurt people's feelings or saying no for the hell of it. What I mean is this: If something isn't a resounding, fiery YES! for you, it's a no. Take that in for a moment. Unless you are over-the-moon excited to say yes, it is a no. Sure, there are things that you'll do that you don't necessarily want to—washing the dishes, waking up early, changing diapers, filing taxes. But for the most part, following your heart and becoming self-focused is a fundamental part of healing. Yes, that is scary. Growth usually means change and change is scary. Yes, it might rub people the wrong way. Yes, it might mean shedding old relationships, friends, or circumstances. But only by listening to our soul's desires do we actually get to where we need to be. It is absolutely necessary to become self-focused in order to grow. Once I realized that becoming self-focused isn't taking away from others but, rather, inspiring others to do the same, it changed the game. Shining your light as brightly as you can inspires others to do the same.

Listen to Life Cravings

I was once asked, if we listen to what our body is craving, won't we be eating junk food for the rest of our lives? That was very revealing, for two reasons. One, cravings have come to mean only "naughty" things or guilty pleasures. But what we are truly craving has nothing to do with a snack drawer or what's in our freezer. Cravings are not confined to salt-and-vinegar chips and gelato. I'm talking about LIFE CRAVINGS. The huge aha moment for me was not so much when I learned

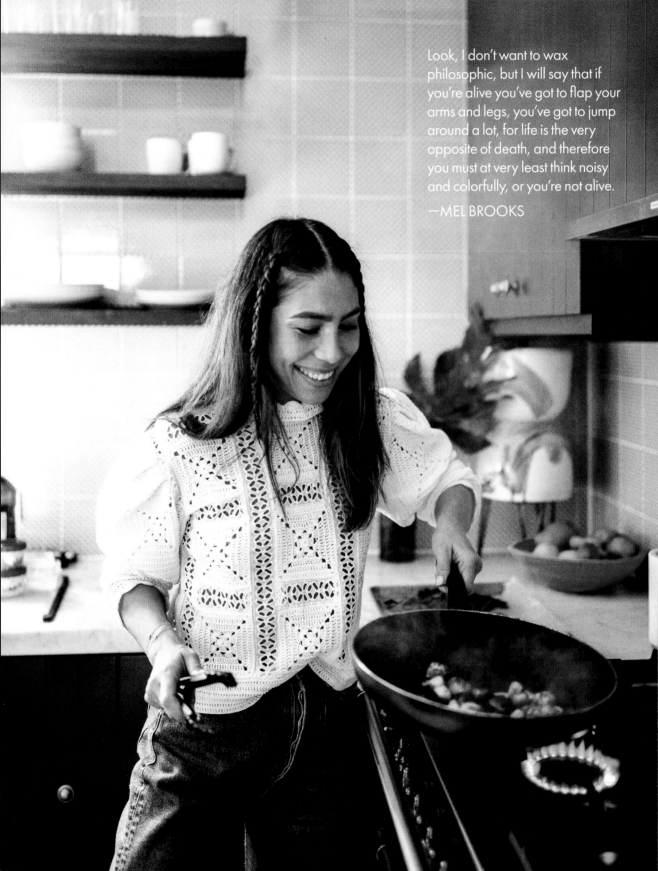

Look, I don't want to wax philosophic, but I will say that if you're alive you've got to flap your arms and legs, you've got to jump around a lot, for life is the very opposite of death, and therefore you must at very least think noisy and colorfully, or you're not alive.

—MEL BROOKS

how to food-combine or switched to a plant-based diet. It was when I began following my heart and what I truly desired in my life. By taking an inventory of what truly makes us happy, we will begin to uncover where our true cravings lie, and they are almost never related to food—unless you want to become a chef!

When we begin to feed our soul what it's been craving, our emotional attachment to food disappears, almost without any effort. If you have battled emotional eating for most of your life (as I had), this is a revelation. It means that we do not have to "fix" our emotional attachment to food, we simply need to feed our emotional desires. I'll say that again. To heal emotional eating, we must feed our emotional needs. Which brings me to the second implication of that innocent question: Once we allow ourselves some freedom, we will never be able to stop. Think about that. We have been told to believe (and you'd better believe we have been told—by television shows, newscasters, magazines, the fashion industry, Hollywood, and now social media) that we cannot be trusted. We, who were born with bodies, spirits, and minds of our own, must be told what to eat, how much of it to eat, and when to eat it. Otherwise, we are lost souls and, left to our own devices, we will curl up in a snack drawer, bingeing our way to oblivion. This is the undercurrent of fear that keeps us from saying yes to our desires and cravings. But if we shine a light on it, that image of us bloated on junk food seems silly, doesn't it? We can be allowed to trust ourselves again, if only we would give ourselves the chance.

Find Your South Beach

Many years ago, I worked with a holistic food coach who once asked me when I feel my happiest and lightest. I answered, "When I'm on vacation in Miami." It was and is true. I love South Beach. To me, it means sunshine, swimming in the ocean, going for jogs on the boardwalk alongside the beach, and delicious healthy food. Whenever I am there, the energy of the city and people inspires me to be more active, eat tons of healthy food, jump in the ocean, run with the sea breeze in my hair, and really not think twice about how much or what I'm eating. I told my coach I crave being in Miami when I'm not there. She told me that when I talked about going to Miami, my demeanor and energy instantly lightened and brightened. She asked, how can you incorporate little things in your daily life to get the feeling of being in Miami, even when you're in New York City? That was a game changer for me. I realized it was not just the city but my own approach to myself that changed in Miami, and I could definitely use that same outlook at home. So I joined a light-filled gym that blasted dance music, made a Miamian smoothie every morning, and made sure I did one self-care thing for myself every day, as I do when I'm in Miami. Everything changed for me simply because I changed my outlook.

When we seek, and I mean actively seek, ways to incorporate more joy in our lives, we start to understand the value of feeling good and we continue to seek more of it.

ON HUNGER

Now let's dive into the eating part of intuitive eating. Once we get in tune with our spirit, we can finally listen to our body's messages and we can start to decipher the signals. The truth is that no matter how many green smoothies, chia seed concoctions, and kale salad we ingest, until we can distinguish true physical hunger from trying to fill an emotional void, we will always be confused about the role nourishing food has in our lives. When I took the time to truly notice my body's cues and my spirit's cues, I began to be able to give my body what it needed. So, before we delve into all the delicious recipes, let's ask ourselves what real hunger feels like.

Identify Spiritual Hunger

We know that when we're feeling false hunger, we are looking for something other than food. When it hits, take a couple of minutes, close your eyes, and ask yourself what you are truly craving.

Let's say you're at the office and your boss is throwing nonstop demands your way, and you reach for a snack in your desk and bury your head in your work. Let's take a moment. Are you hungry? Do you have an urgent need to eat? Is there nothing you can think about other than that snack? Here is where I would ask you to pause. Close your eyes and take five deep breaths. Think "I am calm" as your breathe in, "I am at peace" as you breathe out. Maybe what you are truly craving is a break, or maybe to leave this job. That's okay. Even if you can't fulfill that true desire in that exact moment, just naming it will bring relief. Acknowledge the pain/desire/feeling, and that will feel good. Still want the snack? Go for

it. Intuitive eating is not about ignoring our physical cravings, even if they are intertwined with emotion. Emotions will always be linked with food and that is a beautiful thing. The mistake that so many "diets" make is trying to eliminate emotion from eating—the food-as-fuel gig. Yes, food is fuel. But it is so much more than that. And when we begin to honor our feelings and truly sit with them, then we are able to enjoy food not only for its nutrients but also for the joy it gives us. The reason I work with food is because I've derived joy from food ever since I was a child. But the key element is to pause to register our feelings and continue from a place of presence and mindfulness.

As we say yes to our cravings, we will relearn the signifiers of feeling full and our natural inclination to stop. But because we have been saying no to ourselves for so long, in the beginning we may not know how to stop, and that's okay. Knowing when to stop is different from depriving ourselves. The issue is, because we've deprived ourselves for so long, our natural inclination to stop when we're full is compromised. We must relearn those cues.

Spiritual Hunger Cues

Spiritual hunger is different from actual hunger. It signals a craving deep within our soul, but perhaps we are too disconnected from it or too afraid to recognize it for what it is and we sometimes identify it as real hunger. Some examples of spiritual hunger include:

- BOREDOM
- LONELINESS
- SADNESS
- STRESS
- INSOMNIA

Physical Hunger Cues

Physical hunger is the signal that our bodies need energy and food to survive. It is an important and essential human and animal survival trait. For as long as I can remember, I've been told to fear hunger. Diet and even mainstream culture has long told us to be prepared: Eat small meals throughout the day to sustain our energy and never to get "too" hungry. Have a satiating breakfast in the morning to "prevent" hunger or overeating later, even if we are not hungry when we wake. All these instructions are telling us to fear our own intuition and fear hunger. What flipped it for me was welcoming hunger as a loving sign from my body, not treating it as a problem. It's simply a signal. When we are tired, we sleep. When we are stressed, we rest. When we are hungry, we eat. We don't need to "trick" our body into not being hungry, we should simply go with the flow and listen to our body.

Examples of physical hunger include:

- A GENTLE URGENCY TO EAT RIGHT AT THIS MOMENT
- AN EMPTY STOMACH
- A GROWLING STOMACH
- INABILITY TO THINK OF ANYTHING BUT FOOD IN THAT MOMENT

As for when real hunger hits? Rejoice! I've learned to welcome real hunger with open arms because that's when you can truly enjoy what food has to offer. Let's be clear, I am not advising you to stretch beyond your limits or to not eat when you are hungry. It is the exact opposite. I am inviting you to listen to your body and lean into its cues. And for many, this may be the first time. I know

now that if I'm feeling peckish but not truly hungry, I'd rather wait because I want to be able to enjoy my meal to the fullest, because that is when food tastes the best. If you are mindlessly snacking all day, how will you ever truly savor each bite? This is why I don't subscribe to the ideas of eating six small scheduled meals a day or doing major meal prepping at the beginning of the week. Yes, being prepared is key (see The Body Harmony Kitchen on page 47), but we deny ourselves the joy of eating what we want when we want it if we're overprepared. We deny our intuition by telling ourselves days in advance what we are going to eat or how much. The goal of this book is to return to that childhood joy of eating for true pleasure. Remember, joy comes first in intuitive eating, and spontaneity is the gatekeeper of joy.

Indulge

In order to relearn the cues of physical hunger, we must let ourselves indulge. For so long, we have conditioned ourselves to steer clear of indulgence. Years of dieting and depriving have the potential to create a ravenous energy within ourselves that we feel cannot be trusted. And maybe we can't trust it. If we have said no to [insert "scary" food here] for so long, it becomes all we want. When we sit down and allow ourselves to actually have those things, we binge. It is important, first and foremost, to forgive ourselves. We cannot be blamed. How could we? It's a natural result of deprivation. Next, I ask you to say yes to those indulgences.

It may sound groundbreaking and even counterintuitive, but I encourage you to say yes to everything and anything you want. Forget about what's plant-based or not, what's processed or whole. If you want it, have it. I know it's scary. I know it's terrifying. But as long as we are mindful of our choices and are fully present in the moment, as we begin to say yes to those cravings, their power over us diminishes. In turn, we become empowered to make the choices that make us feel good. What happens is no less than a miracle. The said indulgence no longer has a hold on us and we are no longer using food as a way to reward or punish ourselves, which intrinsically separates us from food as a source of nourishment and joy. There are no more "good days" or "cheat days"; we stop assigning food to a category whose value we then attach to ourselves. We use food for its true purposes instead: simply to nourish and to enjoy. And what a blessing that becomes.

Be Mindful

The first step to making food a celebration and not a drug is becoming mindful. At each meal or snack, try eating without looking at your phone or the television. The tastes and textures and nuances of every ingredient—fruit, vegetable, spice, and grain—come alive in our mouths and we start to understand our taste buds and what makes our bodies and spirits sing. "Sitting in mindfulness, both our bodies and minds can be at peace and totally relaxed," says Thich Nhat Hanh. "In mindfulness, one is not only restful and happy, but alert and awake." When we numb ourselves with outside distractions, food becomes a means to an end. We seek food to make us full so we don't have to think or feel anything.

Part of my healing meant enjoying foods, all foods, in public. I reveled in ordering whatever I wanted in order to mindfully enjoy that food, not shrouded in shame, but out in the open. And as I did so, the food's emotional power decreased.

Learn How to Pivot

Here's the thing. Life happens. People who naturally follow their intuition are grounded and yet often able to pivot and be resilient when challenges come their way. Losing a job, ending a relationship, losing a loved one, getting pregnant, going through a life change or a pandemic—these things will turn you upside down. Being able to go with the flow is an essential tool that you can master only by listening to your intuition.

Still, there are traumatic moments when the last thing you want to do is tap in. During those intense moments, it's more important than ever to give ourselves grace and the space to just be. One of those moments for me was when my daughter, Sea, was born. Instead of going home the next day as she was meant to, she was kept on oxygen in newborn intensive care for seven days, because of complications. It was the hardest week of my life. Two of those days were taken up by tests for quite serious issues. I couldn't feel. I had just given birth and I could not feed my baby. I no longer even had a bed to sleep in, since my stay at the hospital had ended. I slept on two folding chairs in the waiting room, hoping for an answer and pumping syringes full of colostrum that I would drop into Sea's mouth in the space between the breathing tubes. This was a moment when I disconnected from my body because I had to. Trauma will do that to you. We must allow ourselves the grace to do that. There will be a time to return; there will be time to heal.

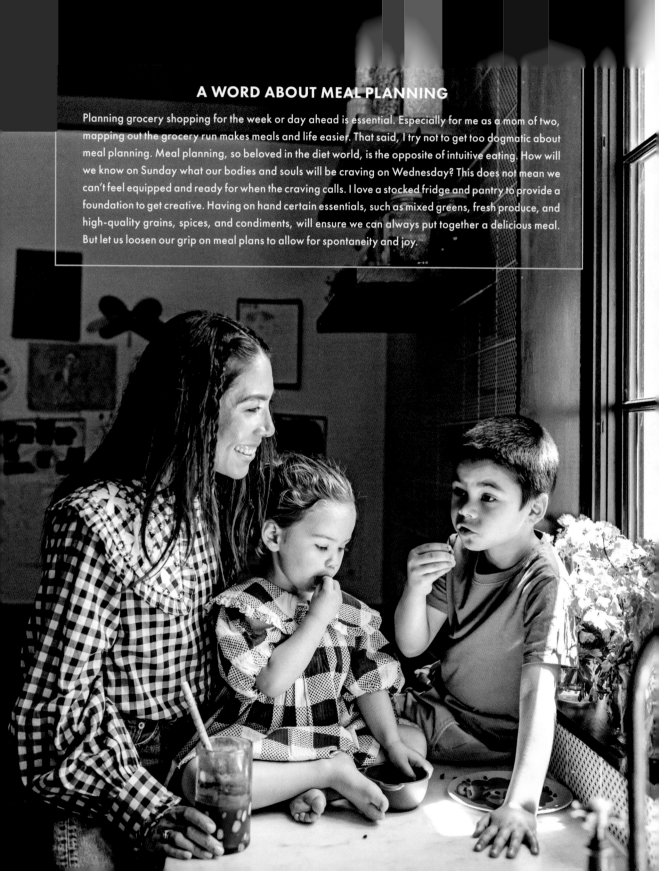

A WORD ABOUT MEAL PLANNING

Planning grocery shopping for the week or day ahead is essential. Especially for me as a mom of two, mapping out the grocery run makes meals and life easier. That said, I try not to get too dogmatic about meal planning. Meal planning, so beloved in the diet world, is the opposite of intuitive eating. How will we know on Sunday what our bodies and souls will be craving on Wednesday? This does not mean we can't feel equipped and ready for when the craving calls. I love a stocked fridge and pantry to provide a foundation to get creative. Having on hand certain essentials, such as mixed greens, fresh produce, and high-quality grains, spices, and condiments, will ensure we can always put together a delicious meal. But let us loosen our grip on meal plans to allow for spontaneity and joy.

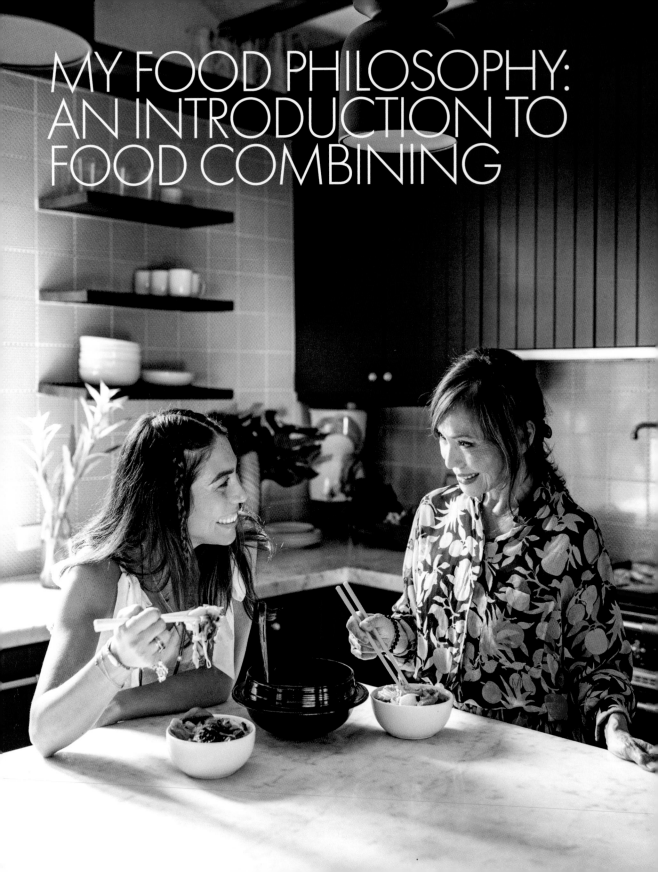

MY FOOD PHILOSOPHY: AN INTRODUCTION TO FOOD COMBINING

First Things First

When I first learned about food combining, I was immediately struck by the freedom it gives you. Instead of rules and restrictions, it presents broad principles that you can follow to feel your best. In empowers you to make your own choices based on how you feel. This was incredibly enlightening for me. Up until then, I had never heard of a plan that simply said, take it or leave it, but if you follow these guidelines, you'll probably feel much better. It gives you the power to decide: Does this method of eating make me feel better? For me, the answer was a resounding yes. Food combining helped me better tune in to my body, observe how my body felt, and make small shifts accordingly.

But before you try food combining, it is essential to first follow your gut. I don't mean in a probiotic, prebiotic way. I mean the old-school way. Follow that voice inside (aka your intuition) and do only what speaks to you. In fact, I encourage you to always be your own guide when nourishing your body and soul. This practice will help you trust your body (no one else's) and what it needs first and foremost—before you try this food philosophy, or any philosophy for that matter. The first person you need to learn to listen to is YOU.

Once we learn to eat intuitively and follow our body's signals, it is helpful, I have found, to have a framework of broad principles to help navigate the modern world—particularly the world of wellness in which there are so many contradictory messages. Sometimes we need structure in order to feel empowered. Structure helps move us through those days when we feel stuck and unmotivated. Structure is a point of reference, or "home," that we can stray from or stay close to, as we please.

Think of intuition as our guiding light, and of food combining as a more structured, earthly plan of action.

Some pages of this chapter may not speak to you, or you may like some parts and not relate to the rest. That is fine. The more than one hundred recipes in the second half of the book can be made and enjoyed whether you follow food combining or not. I'm offering principles and options meant to empower you to feel good, not restrict you. When we move from a place of intuition, we are able to translate these principles in a way that serves us best.

What Is Food Combining?

One day, while shopping at Whole Foods, I came across Natalia Rose's *Raw Food Detox Diet* book and was immediately captivated by the simple image of bright bell peppers. Something made me stop and take the book off the shelf. Through that book I discovered food combining and was introduced to my teacher, Gil Jacobs, a colonic therapist who taught me about the benefits of the cleansing life and changed my perspective on what it means to truly nourish ourselves. Though food combining is one of the oldest, most natural ways to eat, I'm usually met with a perplexed face or a barrage of questions when I explain that this is my food philosophy. With the vegan diet, keto diet, paleo diet, and every other diet under the sun rampant in the health community, food combining has remained elusive, even in the so-called wellness world, and yet, in my experience, it's the most effective lifestyle, when coupled with intuitive eating.

To boil it down to a couple of sentences, food combining is a way to eat and nourish yourself to optimize digestion, energy, mood, and vitality. By combining certain types of foods and consciously not combining others, we allow the body to easily digest natural foods, assimilate them into our body, and release them.

What makes food combining different is that it's not so much about what we are eating as it is about how we eat so not to interfere with our body's natural ability to heal. The time our bodies take to digest different foods varies. For instance, the time it takes to digest a bowl of ripe cantaloupe is much shorter than the time it takes to digest a sub sandwich. You've certainly experienced that. After eating a heavy meal, we are usually more tired than we are after a light meal, as our body is working overtime to digest that meal. In food combining, we honor the body's work and the time it takes to digest the food, thus optimizing energy and vitality.

The fun thing about food combining? You immediately feel it. Like, immediately. When we eat intuitively, we follow how our bodies feel. So you could say that food combining, with its effects that are rapidly perceptible in our bodies, is the ultimate intuitive eating method. You could show me case study after case study to prove why a certain diet or a certain food works best, but if I don't feel the shift in my body immediately, I probably won't stick with it for long. When we make some slight adjustments in keeping with food combining principles—eating light to heavy, consciously pairing certain foods, increasing consumption of whole, natural plant-based foods—we can actually feel the energy shift.

"While there is a myriad of different names for modern diseases in medical literature, there is really just one core cause of all these imbalances: clogging of the cells and pathways due to the accumulation of inappropriate matter left behind," writes Natalia Rose in her book *Detox for Women*. "When substances are consumed that are not easily digested and passed through the human body, they leave residue behind. Once the cells are contaminated by this old matter the healthy microbes in the cells develop into unhealthy, antagonistic bacteria and yeast." We see the consequences in weight gain, acne, body odor, yeast infections, and potentially more serious chronic and autoimmune issues. Shifting to a more plant-based and food-combined diet allows our bodies to gently detoxify by ridding the body of waste, old and new, so that we can claim our bodies back.

In other words, our vitality is dependent on flow. More flow = more vitality. This is not a new idea—many ancient civilizations attach great value to life force. In Asia, it's called *chi*; in Ayurvedic medicine, *prana*; in Polynesia, *mana*; in Hinduism, *Shakti*. Food combining helps keep the body in flow—unobstructed—and in harmony.

WHAT IS LIFE FORCE?

Life force is a term I learned many years ago from my teacher, health guru Gil Jacobs, to describe the energy certain foods have to help our bodies not only survive but thrive. Other cultures use the terms *prana* or *chi* for the vital energy that propels life. Raw salads are packed with *life force*. By becoming in tune with what fed my *life force*, namely, fruit, vegetable juices, and salads, I've been able to seek out these foods with joy rather than regard them as a punishment or dreary element of a diet.

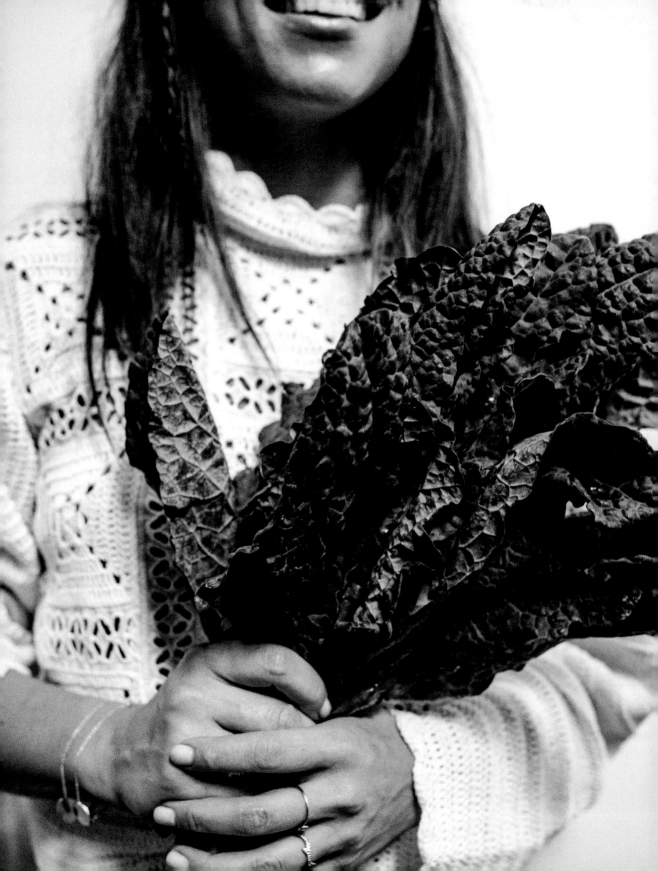

THE PRINCIPLES

Think of these principles more as a road map. Dip in and out as you please, always keeping in mind what serves you in your life at that moment. But when I adhere to them closely, I feel my best.

Fast-Digesting Foods

Remember the idea of chi and prana? In order to cultivate more energy, we focus on fast-digesting foods as much as possible so that our bodies are not burdened with devoting energy to digesting all the time. Examples of fast-digesting, or "quick exit," foods include all fruits, fruit and vegetable juices, raw leafy greens, and raw vegetables. Coffee, though not nutrient-dense, is also a fast-digesting food. We enjoy lighter, raw fruits, juices, and smoothies earlier in the day, typically in the morning, as they are digested and leave the body quickly, allowing us to retain energy to conquer the day. That is not to say we should be having only these foods. Rather, it is important to be aware and observe which foods fuel energy and which deplete us of energy.

Slow-Digesting Foods

Foods that take slightly longer to digest include cooked non-starchy vegetables like steamed broccoli, sautéed spinach, and roasted asparagus. As we know, cooked vegetables are super nutrient-dense. They have an important role because the longer time the body needs to digest them means that they slow down cleansing. They also ground and satiate us. When we incorporate more cooked vegetables and grains in our diet, our bodies can cleanse slowly, which is not only more enjoyable but also gentler on our bodies, which can mean a more effective cleanse. Keep in mind: We are looking for consistency and long-term joy and harmony.

Further down the hierarchy of heavier foods come starchy vegetables. Think of yams, baked potatoes, plantains, winter squashes. Then come grains—quinoa, millet, wild rice, brown rice, white rice, sourdough bread, pastas. Then come legumes, peas, chickpeas, and lentils. Finally comes the heaviest food, animal protein—dairy, fish, eggs, poultry, red meat—which takes the longest to digest. In food combining, we enjoy these heavier foods late in the day when our body is gearing up to rest.

When I began this lifestyle in my early twenties, I had about one-quarter of the energy I do now. And by simply food combining, I noticed radical change. Of course, when we apply food combining principles through a lens of intuitive eating, if we feel we want a heavier breakfast one day, or are traveling and want to indulge in, say, paella or a croissant au chocolat, we listen to our bodies and souls—and go ahead and celebrate. The more we listen, however, the more acutely we comprehend our bodies, and we will more often than not make the choices that cause our bodies to feel good and thrive.

Structure Your Meals Light to Heavy

When we understand that we digest raw foods the fastest, and cooked, dense foods slowly, the order of foods becomes super important but not at all complicated. To maximize energy, we simply start our days off with our lightest meal (juices, smoothies, fruit) and end with our heaviest (big salad and cooked food of choice!). Within meals, we aim to have a large raw salad first to help digest the heavier meal. Let's take lunch. We want to begin with a large leafy green salad—yes, because our body digests it the most quickly, but also because raw leafy greens are alive and packed with live enzymes that can help break down the heavier foods to come. What's great is that we are accustomed to ordering a salad before our meal so it's actually quite a natural way to eat. The more I became aware of my meals, I found that when I skip the salad before a cooked meal, I don't feel as energetic as I do when I preface my meal with raw greens. Try it and see how you feel!

Choose a Protein or a Starch at Each Meal, But Not Both

In his book *Become Younger*, Dr. Norman W. Walker, one of the fathers of juicing and food combining and the inventor of the Norwalk Juicer, writes, "When carbohydrates are eaten during the same meal in which any protein is included, we have a serious chemical situation to contend with. When we eat incompatible mixtures of food, such as meat and potatoes, bread and jam, fruit and sugar, a great deal of fermentation takes place and the formation of gas is unbelievable." This was a major aha moment for me when I began to observe how combining these foods made me feel after a meal. I usually chalked it up to eating too much or too fast, or to certain foods not "agreeing" with me. When I began to experiment with focusing separately on grain- or starch-based meals and protein-based meals, I was shocked at how great I felt almost immediately. That is why food combining is such a tactile method—you feel it right away! So, in order to aid digestion and expedite the process of food leaving the body, we try not to mix food groups, which brings me to the next principle.

In food combining we aim to choose one dense food—protein or starch—at a time. When you pick one category, either starch (grains, starchy root veggies) or protein (dairy, meats, seafood), your body can more efficiently digest what it's being fed. If you are vegan, you're taking away much of the guesswork since you don't have to think much about pairing protein and starches. If you're not fully plant-based, you can enjoy your wild salmon, roast chicken, or grass-fed steak paired with non-starchy vegetables like spinach or broccoli rabe—just nix the potato. They mean it when they call meat and potatoes "stick-to-your-ribs" meals.

Order Matters

While plant-based whole foods have the power to radically heal, when they are put in the body matters just as much than their mere consumption. But just because they are "plant-based" does not mean they are inherently healing. In college, I was a "junk food vegan," strictly vegan but mainly subsisted on "chik" nuggets, frozen bean burritos and Zone bars. It was hugely eye-opening for me to learn the true healing power of plant foods lie not in the mere omission of animal-based product but in their mostly pure, raw, untouched state. When we increase our intake of alkaline, nutrient-dense, water-containing juices and foods (read: fruits and vegetables), they can help pull waste up (and, ideally, out) of our bodies through elimination and sweat.

But, if these healing foods awaken waste but that waste cannot leave the body, the result can be pain, gas, bloating, and the like.

"The formation of gas is a natural chemical action whereby matter is converted from a solid or a liquid into a gaseous state," writes Dr. Norman Walker. "When we eat or drink food in the wrong combinations, the gas which is generated by the fermentation and putrefaction of such food can cause a terrific amount of pressure in any part of the digestive tract."

THE CATEGORIES

Now that we understand the grand scheme of food combining, we need to know about certain categories that different types of food fall into. Understanding their role helps us when making combinations.

Green Juice

This is the core of the Body Harmony lifestyle. Unadulterated, raw fruits and vegetables are the life-giving force for all human beings. Think of green juice or a green smoothie as your daily nutrient boost and your foundation for the day ahead. With two toddlers, both of whom have their picky phases, I turn to a green juice as a way of ensuring they will get the nutrients and vitamins they need. Vegetable juice, particularly juice extracted from green leafy vegetables, is one of the most healing

> ### RAW JUICE VERSUS PASTEURIZED JUICE
>
> Remember, not all juice is created equal. The swampy contents of the bottle collecting dust in your local deli's fridge is a different beast from the juice you make at home. "Juices must be RAW in order to be vital and of constructive value," writes Norman Walker. "When juices have been canned, processed, preserved, or pasteurized, their life principle has been extinguished and their vital value destroyed." This is why I absolutely recommend investing in a home juicer. Juicing at home is quick, it's cheaper and more sustainable than buying juice elsewhere, and you can ensure that the juice is fresh! Cold-press or centrifugal? For me, the type that is easier or more efficient to incorporate in your life is the one to go with.

substances, if not the most healing, that we can nourish ourselves with.

"Drinking the juice of green plants (romaine lettuce, spinach, collard greens, etc.) . . . renew[s] every cell it reaches," writes Natalia Rose in *Detox for Women*. "It cleans the blood through its rich alkalinity, near bio-identical makeup to hemoglobin, delivers the most absorbable form of minerals, floods the body with fresh Life Force Energy, and makes you feel absolutely fresh and energetic."

That said, when a person shocks their system by going from a mainstream diet to a juice cleanse, they might get headaches, feel bloated, and break out. This is not the juice's doing; rather, the body, trying to eliminate, is not able to release. That is the detoxifying power that green juice has. Green juice has a medicinal purpose—to heal and pull out. If we are not able to efficiently eliminate, however, the waste can be reabsorbed into our system and make us feel worse. This is why, in food combining, we are very strategic in having green juice or a green smoothie at the beginning of the day. Our vessels are empty then, and we are able to absorb and assimilate the energy-rich chlorophyll packed in raw leafy greens. By drinking green, we do not expend the energy needed to chew and digest foods—and, as Natalia Rose pictured it, we infuse our blood with the energy of the sun. So it is essential, when introducing more juices and salads into the body, to temper the cleanse with slower-digesting foods like cooked vegetables, squash, and high-quality grains, and to follow the rules of food combining.

The best time to have your green juice? In the morning, on an empty stomach. Since green juice assimilates into the body quickly and exits the body quickly, it is ideal to have it first thing. But it is perhaps most important that it taste good.

Remember, joy comes first. I warn juicing newbies that you typically get a groan or grimace when you mention green juice—as if it's meant to taste like a green, swampy mess. On the contrary! When mixed with tart green apples, lemons, and ginger, it tastes better than lemonade!

Raw Salads

Salads can be a beautiful way to incorporate more nutrients, prebiotic fiber, and live enzymes in your life—all of which will feed your energy and make you feel vibrant. Yes, abundant salads are gorgeous, plentiful, and delicious, but most importantly, they are arming you with the natural plant-based digestive enzymes that help break down the heavier meal to come. As Gil Jacobs puts it, salads are our "bulletproof vest" for what comes next. What he means is that raw, living vegetables, particularly leafy greens and sprouts, are packed with enzymes to help your gut digest food and absorb nutrients. Without raw vegetables, cooked foods can sit in the gut and be left to ferment—and remember, the secret to vitality is elimination.

"Fresh foods are considered good for the body because, aside from containing many enzymes, they are not oxidized," writes Dr. Hiromi Shinya in *The Enzyme Factor*. "Oxidation occurs when matter bonds with oxygen and 'rusts.' Free radicals are created when these oxidized foods enter the body . . . free radicals are known to destroy DNA cells, causing cancer and many other health problems." Translation: We aim to eat plenty of raw vegetable juices, freshly squeezed fruit juices, whole fruits, leafy greens, and salads—as much as possible to nourish your body to, yes, survive but most importantly thrive.

An easy rule of thumb? Start each cooked meal with a leafy green salad. Simple enough, right? Luckily our culture supports starting meals with salad so it's an easy practice, especially when you're dining out. Just make sure the salads aren't mixed with other things like fruits, nuts, and seeds that might hamper digestion and collide with your cooked dinner.

When I was first told that just eating a raw salad at every meal before eating cooked food would massively change my digestion, I was thrilled. That seemed like the easiest thing ever! And it was. It also increased my energy tenfold. It's one of the reasons I love this lifestyle so much.

Neutral Cooked Vegetables

Neutral cooked vegetables (sautéed spinach, steamed broccoli, roasted asparagus, and more) are our secret weapon for living in harmony. As I've mentioned before, it is key to transition slowly into a more cleansing life. If you were raised on meat and potatoes, mac and cheese, and Lucky Charms, it could potentially be detrimental to go from that to living on raw juices and fruits. Shocking the system with only juices or raw vegetables could cause more harm and also make you feel deprived and resent the lifestyle entirely, or, worse, reignite old deprivation patterns. Cooked vegetables are incredibly healing and grounding, especially when our bodies need to slow down, enjoy, and indulge.

After graduating from college, I dabbled in being a raw foodie, which was all the rage in the early aughts. There was a very fancy and trendy restaurant I frequented with stunning dishes to match. But after leaving a three- to four-course meal of raw salad, nut-based lasagna, and mint-chip cashew ice cream, I felt exhausted, heavy, and uncomfortable. Though

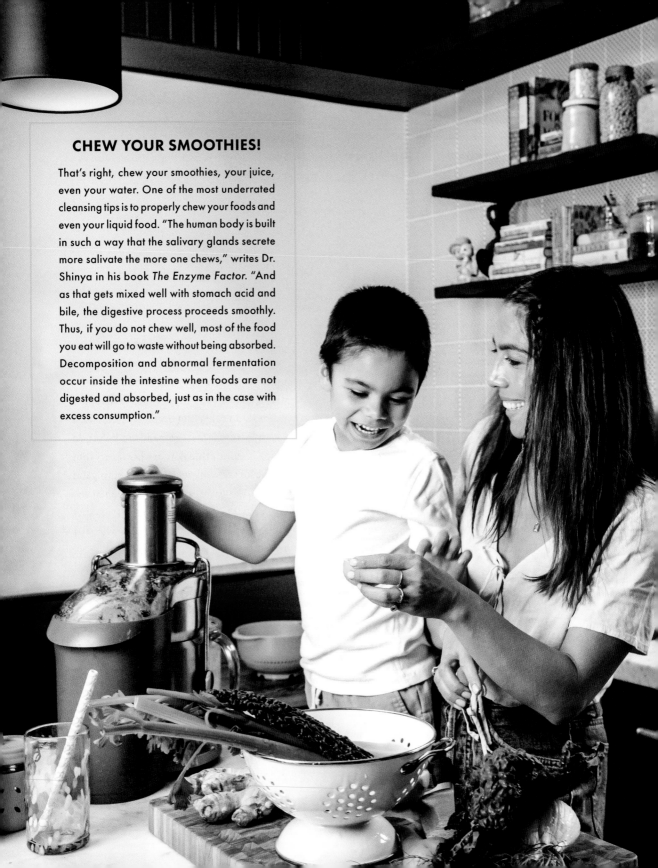

CHEW YOUR SMOOTHIES!

That's right, chew your smoothies, your juice, even your water. One of the most underrated cleansing tips is to properly chew your foods and even your liquid food. "The human body is built in such a way that the salivary glands secrete more salivate the more one chews," writes Dr. Shinya in his book *The Enzyme Factor*. "And as that gets mixed well with stomach acid and bile, the digestive process proceeds smoothly. Thus, if you do not chew well, most of the food you eat will go to waste without being absorbed. Decomposition and abnormal fermentation occur inside the intestine when foods are not digested and absorbed, just as in the case with excess consumption."

all these foods were alive, they were incredibly dense. Once I learned that actually easing up on raw foods and incorporating simply cooked vegetables into my diet would not only increase my energy but improve my digestion, I was all in.

Starchy Vegetables and Legumes

Potatoes and winter squash are some of my favorite foods on the planet. Whenever I incorporate them in a meal, I immediately feel grounded, nourished, and comforted. I like to call Japanese yam nature's candy! In Asian cultures, starchy vegetables have an important place in warming the body, particularly in the colder months. I find I am more drawn to these heavier vegetables as the temperatures dip. Again, as you become more present and observant, you'll notice how your body naturally gravitates toward seasonal things.

Legumes are a funny thing. Technically, they are both a starch and a protein, which makes them a bit of an imperfect food. You know the old adage, "Beans, beans they make you . . ." You know the rest. The reason is, since they combine a starch and protein, they can create gas in the body. That said, I really enjoy beans and lentils and think they are wonderfully helpful when transitioning to a more plant-based diet. You'll find them in the book with starchy vegetables, since I believe they are easier digested with grains rather than proteins (since animal protein takes so long to digest, adding legumes on top can amount to a very dense meal). However, integrate them how you like or not at all!

What about Protein?

Although the recipes in this book are fully plant-based, I fully support making your own choice to incorporate protein as you see fit within the food combining framework. In fact, sometimes when I'm craving a piece of wild salmon, grilled halloumi cheese or organic roast chicken, I'll have it but make sure to preface it with a big green salad and plenty of non-starchy vegetables. I always say, I feel better ordering like that at an Italian trattoria or French bistro than going to a raw foodie or vegan restaurant when they put every nut, seed, grain and legume into one dish and I end up feeling more lethargic than I would having grass-fed steak and greens. This is why I am not a fan of the fake meats and cheeses on a regular basis. They are fun to try now and then but certainly not health foods by any stretch. If your choice to be vegan is ecological and/or ethical, more power to you! Just be mindful that what most you are eating are whole vegetables, grains and not too much of the processed stuff. That bring us back to the age-old question of what role protein plays in a balanced diet. Yes, protein is essential but the emphasis on animal protein, in my opinion, is a bit skewed. "Animal proteins are considered good quality proteins since they contain all of the essential amino acids. It is because of this that modern nutritionists tell you to have animal proteins every day," writes Dr. Hiromi Shinya. "But plant proteins also contain many, although not all of the essential amino acids. Grains, cereals, legumes, vegetables, mushrooms, fruits and sea vegetables all contain many amino acids. Many people are surprised when they are told that 37% of nori (dried seaweed) is protein, but many people know that the sea vegetable kelp is a treasure house of amino acids." When I keep my diet extremely varied, rich with raw and cooked vegetables, plant-based fats, legumes, hearty grains and various seaweeds, I not only feel satiated but incredibly grounded and energized. And though I am not completely vegan, I do find the plant-based life wonderfully abundant in its offerings and almost never think about how I "get my protein."

Soaking grains in water for 3 hours to overnight helps make them more digestible.

Grains

Grains, or "carbs," have been vilified for years, but when I began to lovingly incorporate them in my meals, it was the ultimate act of self-care since they can be so healing and grounding, particularly if we are focusing on high-quality anti-inflammatory grains. I also find them incredibly helpful when you are transitioning to a more plant-based lifestyle. And by the way, I am very happy to live in this transition phase forever. For me, balancing high vitality with indulgence and joy is very important, so I am happy to combine them to achieve body harmony. For me, high-quality grains include sourdough breads, sprouted-grain breads, wild rice, white rice, brown rice, quinoa, kasha, and buckwheat- and rice-based noodles and pastas. When eaten after a raw salad and alongside plenty of cooked vegetables, grains are incredibly grounding and indulgent.

THE JUICES VS. SMOOTHIES DEBATE

While green juice extracts the life force from vegetables and delivers it directly to your bloodstream and cells, green smoothies retain the vegetables' fiber, and so act as a scrubbing worker bee to help facilitate elimination. By blending the greens, you are almost "pre-digesting" the nutrients to help you absorb them with ease. Think of a smoothie as a blended salad, for a gentle detox. And although it's a slower detox than juices, it's still as effective, especially in the beginning of your Body Harmony journey. Remember, transitional detox can be a great help.

If you don't have a juicer, or if it's too expensive to purchase copious amount of produce daily, green smoothies are a great alternative. I call them green juice on training wheels. They also keep overnight in the fridge, whereas juices lose their vitality after a few hours. Just remember to keep protein powders, nuts, seeds, and butters out of smoothies. We've been conditioned to believe that the more you put in your smoothie, the better it will fill you up. But that's all it will do: fill you up and weigh you down. There are so many smoothies these days that mix nuts, oats, butters, and powders, you're almost better off having a green salad and steak! The smoothie recipes in this book are designed to improve, not impede, elimination and digestion.

On Fruit: Eat It Alone, or Leave It Alone

Fruit is one of the cleanest, purest foods you can eat. That said, there is one principle I follow that changed the way I feel toward fruit forever—eat fruit alone, or leave it alone. Why? Fruit is almost all water, and because of that, it is digested faster than any other food. When we eat fruit on an empty stomach, say, in the morning, our bodies are able to assimilate that fruit and use its nutrients and minerals—and the fiber that fruit is packed with is the ultimate natural eliminator. (Remember, flow = vitality.) A good test of this: If you begin to eat fruit on an empty stomach, watch your elimination skyrocket later that day or even immediately.

If, however, we eat fruit after a cooked meal—say, a fruit plate after a big dinner—we ask our bodies to contend with two different digestive processes: the slow digestion of the cooked food and the fast digestion of the fruit. The result? Fermentation, bloating, and discomfort. You probably have experienced this before, when you have a heavy meal and decide to have a "light" dessert, aka the fruit plate, and suddenly you feel an immediate pain in your stomach. This means no more pairing bananas and berries with cereal or oatmeal, and, ideally, no fruits in your almond milk smoothie.

Simply making this one shift—to eating fruit on an empty stomach—is game changing. It also opens up the possibility of enjoying fruit in abundance. We have been told time and again to fear fruit, yet it is the most natural food on earth, put here for human consumption. It would be strange, if not a bit sadistic, if Mother Nature made this glorious sweet-tasting food available if it was actually not good for us.

The issue is not the fruit in and of itself—it is the way we are eating it. What's more, if we have been avoiding a plant-based diet rich in water-containing foods for months or even years, and we shift radically to a mostly raw diet, we are probably going to experience some discomfort. This is because fruit is so cleansing and healing, it will bring up a lot of stuff. Gil Jacobs likens it to a therapy session in which old trauma gets triggered. Usually the therapist will go slowly, not straight to the heart of the issue. It's the same with cleansing. We want to slowly integrate cleansing foods in the right place for an effective, easy cleanse. If you feel you thrive on fruits, begin your day with a heaping plate of your favorite fruits (ideally, seasonal). They will give your body an alkaline boost to ensure better digestion and enzymes for the remainder of the day without overcleansing your system. If you feel fruit is too activating and you don't feel well eating it, leave it alone. Again, we listen to our bodies first and foremost. Nobody is in the driver's seat but you.

Remember, Detox Is Not What Goes In, It's What Comes Out

Now for the big one. One of the greatest misconceptions in the wellness industry, especially in the age of juice bars on every corner, is that juicing or unidentifiable powders we drop into our water are inherently detoxifying. It's not. Detoxing is not what you put in your body, it's what's coming out.

Think of everything you have ever eaten in your life. The Cinnamon Toast Crunch, the Jägermeister shots in college, the McDonald's burgers, the string cheese, the steak frites. Much of this food was certainly fun, but it was not necessarily ideal for human consumption, and so our body cannot eliminate all of it on its own. Sure, we eliminate, but our bodies were not designed to digest Lunchables, Flaming Hot Cheetos, and Gushers (if you were into that kind of thing, which I was). Whatever our bodies cannot digest can remain in our body, and as years pass, waste piles up, and it eventually leads to weight gain, premature aging,

fatigue, overall discomfort, and, possibly, disease.

As Walker puts it, "Coupled with the failure to nourish the body with the proper type and kind of food in the past, the retention of waste matter in the system positively helps the development of ailments and the speedy approach of the appearance of old age." Embarking on a juice cleanse or going vegan does not itself cure us of years of vice. But it can act as a sort of Windex to ease the removal of waste. Then we need the Junk Luggers to haul it all out. As Jacobs says, "The biggest misconception is that fasting makes you healthier. Completion of a juice fast does not ensure success; it just means that potential for cleansing is present. If you do it too wrong and too long you can make yourself deathly ill."

When we consciously food combine and increase our raw greens before a cooked meal, our digestion can improve immediately, as can our elimination. That is because when we increase our intake of alkaline, raw foods, we increase enzymes and fiber. You will find many juice, smoothie, and

---

A WORD ON ORGANIC FRUIT AND SEASONALITY

We must not forget that the fruit our indigenous ancestors enjoyed centuries ago is a far cry from the pristine hybrid produce available in most supermarkets. I love fruit in abundance, but it's not as simple as we'd like it to be. Today, many fruits are genetically modified to look nice and taste good. It's important to seek, as much as we can, organic, local, non-GMO fruits that are truly mineral rich and that our bodies can recognize. Sure, it's fun to eat a pink pineapple now and then and indulge in seedless watermelon during the summer, but keep in mind that these are not naturally occurring fruits and can lead to a sugar crash. One good rule of thumb is to maximize seasonality when eating fruits (the same goes for vegetables). When a fruit or vegetable is in season, it is at its highest nutrient content. It also tastes best too. The body is no fool. It has been designed to enjoy what is most nutrient-beneficial. The problem is that we have dulled our senses with genetically modified, artificial flavor and seasoning such that we don't even remember the simple joy derived from an apple in the fall, winter squash in the winter, or a bowl of peaches, plums, and apricots in the summer. Sure, I love avocados and lemons year-round, but when you let the seasons and local abundance guide your meals, you can watch your vitality soar.

salad recipes in this book because of their power to cleanse, and I want that process to be as delicious as possible. It is important that we are consistently eliminating through regular bowel movements and sweating, but also incorporating self-care practices that also help us release, whether it be dry brushing, massages, exercising, or yoga—or even what is sometimes considered radical self-care, like enemas, colonics, and infrared saunas. More on that later.

Be Consistent

No matter which of these practices speak to your soul and feel good to your body, whether you take some and leave the rest, consistency is key. Routine and habit are beautiful things when they are coming from a space of intuition. For me, I intuitively know that I thrive on a green juice almost every morning. Some days I want a smoothie instead, some days I want something heartier, but these routines are in place so that I can opt in for what I am feeling in that moment. What we do most days is better than what we do on other days. Forgive yourself when you falter and keep moving.

ON SNACKING

In food combining, it's important to give the body rest between meals to properly digest the food. If we are constantly snacking/grazing, our body is constantly using energy to digest. My focus is eating abundant meals and feeling truly satiated, so I'm not a big snacker! If I am hungry, by all means, I eat, but I usually eat more of the meal that I'm already having rather than a variety of things throughout the day.

The 70/30 Approach

The most important thing to remember is that we are emotional, spiritual human beings and sometimes we crave more than simply a massive kale salad. (At other times, that's all we need.) The memories, the tastes, the fantasy of food—they are all very real things to address. Remember those pastrami on rye dates I had with my dad? I wouldn't give those up for the world. Nor would I give up fresh baguettes with butter and jam in Paris or paella while vacationing in Spain. Or bagels and tofu cream cheese with my kids on the weekend. Those indulgent moments are just as nourishing as a heaping raw salad, and when we dive into those moments with all of our being, we feel whole and nourished. When I live the closest to my own version of body harmony, I strive to eat 70 percent whole, unprocessed fruits and vegetables, while 30 percent of the time I indulge in foods that I crave and that feed the soul, not just the tummy. Joy first.

Exceptions (Intuitive Eating Again!)

There are certain instances when, as we shift to a more plant-based diet, we tend to feel bloated and more tired. Sometimes our naturopath or doctors instruct us to avoid certain fruits and vegetables in order to heal an imbalance. It is important to keep in mind that we are all coming from different places, emotionally, physically, genetically, and geographically. We must always take this into account and listen to ourselves and practitioners who know what works best for us individually when we are not feeling well. In a perfect world we are meant to thrive naturally on whole, unprocessed foods, which for the most part means fruits and vegetables. If there is an adverse reaction to these foods, it is simply a signal that we have some healing to do. If you are dealing with specific limitations due to a medical diagnosis, I suggest you use my recipes as you would like and make substitutions as needed. If you are allergic to a certain vegetable or have been explicitly told to avoid something, use that as a stimulus to make these recipes your own. My hope is that these guidelines empower you to make your own choices that work best for your own life.

On Families and Raising Children

For me, motherhood has been the biggest assignment in letting go, since kids have plans of their own from the get-go, and it's a beautiful lesson in how to cede control and let it flow. Our children are our biggest teachers and, if anything, they are the ones who are most in tune with their bodies and instinctively know when they are hungry and when they are not. It's about striking a balance in providing as many fresh whole-food options as possible and honoring their intuition in the same way we honor ours.

Our first child Jude, went on a fruit and vegetable strike at age four. I had to remind myself, this is my assignment. I must let go of control. I truly believe that children observe us constantly and see the energy we are putting into our food, how we prepare our food, how we enjoy our food, but not necessarily what the food is. Yes, we want them to be able to identify a fruit and a vegetable, but they will get there if we remain consistent, loving, and joyful when nourishing ourselves. As a parent, it is my job to provide options that are as healthy and nourishing as possible but to allow kids to be kids.

At home, we do gently follow food-combining principles but are not dogmatic or rigid about it. Breakfast is usually a green juice—we make a version of our Green Lemonade and keep it sweet enough so it's really delicious—followed by Jude's French Toast. Lunch is an avocado sandwich, apple, and kettle-cooked potato chips, and dinner is usually pasta or veggie fried rice. When they want chicken, they'll have chicken. We'll do chocolate sorbet sundaes and air-popped popcorn on movie Fridays. For me, joy and the beauty of having loving food memories is something I cherish and want to pass on to my children. And I do this with gentle guidance in mind as I want the foods we choose as a family to only support our everyday ease, happiness and growth. When it comes to kids, there is no one size fits all or steadfast rules. I encourage you to use your intuition (yes, again), to make the choices that feel best for your family at a given time, knowing they may shift and change as your family does. I aim to include one green thing or whole vegetable in every meal, whether that is an avocado, chopped cucumber, steamed broccoli, or cauliflower—or even a pickle. I find the one thing or the few things my children will eat and include that in rotation at every meal. If on some days they don't touch it, that's okay; I always keep it as an option on the plate or in the lunch box. If they begin with a green juice in the morning, they'll always have that foundation if they veer off path later in the day.

When you have the best and tastiest ingredients, you can cook very simply and the food will be extraordinary because it tastes like what it is.

—ALICE WATERS, *The Art of Simple Food*

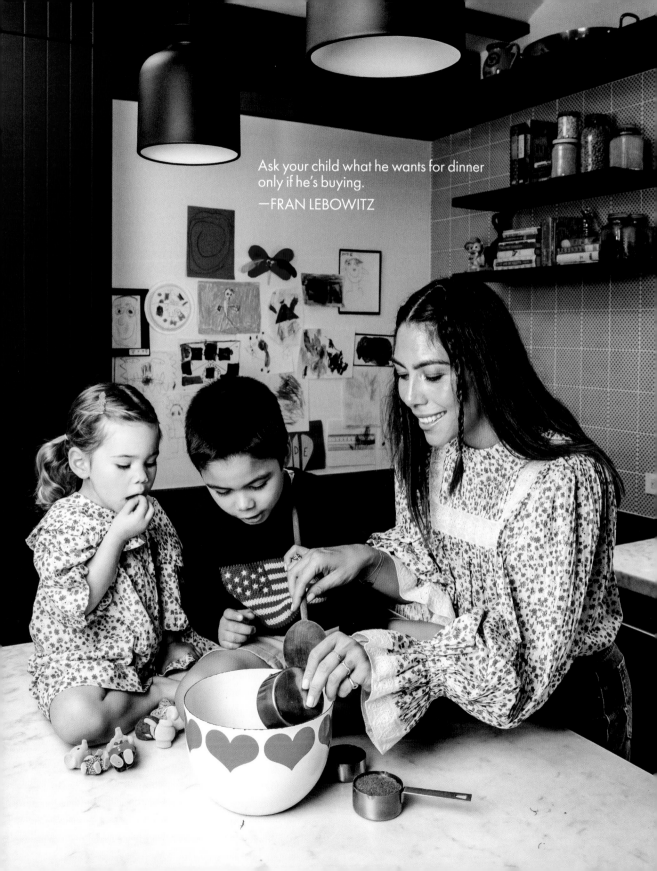

Ask your child what he wants for dinner
only if he's buying.
—FRAN LEBOWITZ

FOOD-COMBINING CHART

FRUITS (EAT THEM ALONE, ON AN EMPTY STOMACH, OR LEAVE THEM ALONE)

Apples, apricots, bananas, berries, citrus fruits (oranges and grapefruit), dragonfruit, grapes, mangoes, melons, papaya, passionfruit, pears, pineapple, stone fruit

NEUTRAL VEGETABLES (PAIR WITH ANYTHING)

All leafy greens (green leaf lettuce, kale, spinach, arugula, dandelion greens, romaine, watercress, bibb, Boston), asparagus, bean sprouts, beets, bok choy, broccoli, broccolini, broccoli rabe, brussels sprouts, cabbage, carrots, cauliflower, celery, chard, collard greens, corn (raw), cucumber, eggplant, endives, garlic, jicama, kale, kohlrabi, mushrooms, okra, olives, onions, radicchio, parsnip, peppers, rutabaga, seaweed, tomatoes, turnips, radicchio, spaghetti squash, water chestnuts, yellow squash, zucchini

NEUTRAL FATS (PAIR WITH ANYTHING)

Avocado oil, coconut oil, cold-pressed olive oil, flax seed oil, grapeseed oil, ghee, grass-fed butter, hemp oil, sesame oil, young coconut

STARCHY VEGETABLES (PAIR WITH NEUTRAL VEGGIES AND FATS AND GRAINS, NOT WITH PROTEINS OR NUTS)

Acorn squash, avocado, butternut squash, corn (cooked), cassava, delicata squash, Japanese yams, kabocha squash, mature coconut, plantains, sweet potatoes, taro, white potatoes, winter squash, yuca

GRAINS (PAIR WITH NEUTRAL VEG AND FAT AND WITH STARCHY VEG)

Amaranth, buckwheat groats, black rice, brown rice, kasha, millet, gluten-free (eggless) pastas, purple rice, quinoa, white rice, sourdough, sprouted grains

PROTEINS (PAIR WITH NEUTRAL VEGGIES AND OTHER PROTEINS, NOT STARCHES OR NUTS)

All animal meats (ideally, grass-fed and hormone-free), cheese (ideally, raw and unpasteurized goat or sheep), eggs (ideally, pasture-raised), fish (ideally, wild and local), milk, yogurt

LEGUMES (COMBINE WITH GRAINS OR PAIR WITH STARCHY VEGETABLES)

Adzuki beans, black beans, borlotti beans, edamame, fava beans, garbanzo beans, kidney beans, lentils, mung beans, peanuts, pinto beans, red beans, red lentils, white beans

NUTS/DRIED FRUIT (COMBINE WITH EACH OTHER OR PAIR WITH NEUTRAL VEGETABLES)

Raw almonds, brazil nuts, cashews, macadamia nuts, walnuts, sunflower seeds, raisins, currants, dried apricots, dried mango

Basic Things to Remember About Food Combining

- Eat fruits, fresh juices, and smoothies alone on an empty stomach.
- Aim not to mix starches and proteins in one sitting.
- Be mindful of oils or cooked fats (I aim for no more than 2 to 4 tablespoons per dish/meal).
- Aim to have a raw salad before every cooked meal.
- Eat light to heavy throughout the day.
- If you're going to splurge, do it at the end of the day.
- Eat when you are hungry.
- Avoid snacking between meals to allow time for your body to digest.

THE BODY HARMONY KITCHEN

WHAT MAKES YOU PREPARED FOR BALANCED MEALS AT ANYTIME IS A PROPERLY STOCKED KITCHEN AND PANTRY. Having a few basic tools and appliances and a well-stocked spice cabinet can mean the difference between a just okay meal and one to remember. Read on to see what's in my artillery.

Kitchen Tools

Though they're not all necessities, there are a few key items that I use day in and day out to speed up meal prep, and they don't take up too much space in my city kitchen.

A GOOD KNIFE

Every respectable home cook needs a sharp butcher's knife for chopping fruits and vegetables; a paring knife to peel veggies and fruits; and a bread knife to wrangle those dense loaves of sourdough.

CAST-IRON SKILLET

Gives the perfect char to any vegetable.

DUTCH OVEN

HIGH-POWERED BLENDER

You want the high-powered ones that will not balk at whipping up creamy smoothies out of four or five rock-hard frozen bananas or making a big batch of aquafaba mayo. Definitely an essential in the Bonberi kitchen!

MINI FOOD PROCESSOR

Ideal for those days when you're not batch-cooking for twelve.

JULIENNE PEELER

To create "zoodles" from zucchini or shaved carrot for textured salads.

NONSTICK NONTOXIC PAN

For dishes like pancakes, French toast, and other "sticky" dishes.

MANDOLIN

When this tool is used correctly, and carefully, it creates the perfect delicate, paper-thin slices of radishes, cucumbers, zucchini, or onion, and even potato chips!

MICROPLANE

Use a Microplane or the fine-holed side of a cheese grater for lemon and lime zest, garlic, or ginger. You'll find many recipes call for "grated" ginger or garlic and the Microplane is perfect for these moments.

STAINLESS-STEEL STEAMER BASKET

I love to pop this in a pot with a little bit of water and steam up veg for a quick dinner with brown rice or to add to salads.

STAINLESS-STEEL FRYING PAN

Unlike the nonstick versions, they teach you how to control heat, which inevitably makes you a better home cook.

RICE MAKER OR SLOW-COOKER

When I was growing up, my Korean mom always had something in the rice cooker. Recently, I've discovered you can also use it for quinoa, millet, and other grains.

TOASTER OVEN

Truth be told, I use my toaster oven more than my regular oven. It does the trick for roasted veggies, broiled fish, sweet potato fries, and, yes, even toast.

DUTCH OVEN

I love my Le Creuset bright orange French ceramic Dutch oven, and it's lasted for years. I make soups, stocks, and stews in it. It's also perfect for boiling pastas, making curries, and even sautéing veggies, and it wears like a dream.

Groceries

These are things I like to have on hand and that are usually stocked in my fridge and pantry at any given time. I always say a stocked kitchen makes for easy on-the-fly meals.

IN THE FRIDGE

PRODUCE

- ARUGULA
- BABY SPINACH
- BEETS
- BELL PEPPERS
- BERRIES
- CARROTS
- CABBAGE
- CELERY
- CHERRIES
- CUCUMBERS
- FENNEL
- FRESH HERBS (CILANTRO, MINT, PARSLEY, BASIL, DILL)
- KALE (CURLY AND LACINATO)
- LEMONS
- MIXED GREENS
- PERSIAN CUCUMBERS
- RADISHES
- ROMAINE
- ZUCCHINI

CONDIMENTS

- BARREL PICKLES (NOT PICKLED IN VINEGAR)
- CAPERS
- DIJON MUSTARD
- HOT SAUCE

- SAUERKRAUT
- VEGAN KIMCHI (TRADITIONAL KIMCHI HAS SHRIMP PASTE OR FISH SAUCE)
- VEGAN OR AQUAFABA MAYO

FRUIT BOWL

- APPLES
- AVOCADOS
- BANANAS (RIPE)
- CHERRY TOMATOES
- MANGOES
- MELONS
- PEARS
- TOMATOES
- STONE FRUITS (IN THE SUMMER)
- SWEET POTATO OR SQUASH

AROMATICS

- GARLIC
- GINGER
- ONIONS
- SHALLOTS
- TURMERIC

IN THE PANTRY

- APPLE CIDER VINEGAR
- AVOCADO OIL
- CELTIC SEA SALT
- DRIED QUINOA
- GLUTEN-FREE PASTA (I LIKE BROWN RICE, RED LENTIL, OR YELLOW PEA PASTAS THE BEST)
- ORGANIC COLD-PRESSED OLIVE OIL
- LEGUMES, DRIED OR JARRED (BLACK BEANS, CHICKPEAS, LENTILS)
- STORE-BOUGHT MARINARA SAUCE

- JARRED OLIVES
- PEPPER MILL
- RICE (BASMATI, BLACK, BROWN, JASMINE, PURPLE)
- 100% BUCKWHEAT SOBA NOODLES
- RICE VERMICELLI NOODLES
- TAMARI SAUCE
- TOASTED SESAME OIL

IN THE FREEZER

- RIPE BANANAS (FOR SMOOTHIES)
- SOURDOUGH BREAD
- SPROUTED EZEKIEL PITAS AND BREAD
- GRAIN-FREE TORTILLAS (I LIKE SIETE)
- FROZEN MANGO (FOR GREEN SMOOTHIES)
- VEGGIE BURGERS (I LIKE HILARY'S AND DR. PRAEGERS)

IN THE SPICE RACK

- CAYENNE PEPPER
- CHILI POWDER
- CUMIN
- DRIED DILL
- GARLIC POWDER
- GARAM MASALA OR CURRY POWDER
- ONION POWDER
- OREGANO
- PAPRIKA
- TURMERIC
- ZA'ATAR

SWEETENERS (NEUTRAL, BUT USE SPARINGLY)

- COCONUT SUGAR
- MAPLE SYRUP
- STEVIA
- RAW HONEY

SPECIALTY INGREDIENTS THAT I USE OFTEN

- SWEET POTATO YAM NOODLES
- MUNG BEAN NOODLES
- MUNG BEANS

A Word on Shopping International or Specialty Markets

Much of the inspiration for my recipes is drawn from my Korean heritage, and I use some specialty ingredients that aren't easily swapped for mainstream alternatives. (You can find rice cakes and sweet potato or mung bean noodles at most Asian grocers or online.) I encourage exploring your local Asian, Indian, African, Latin, and Middle Eastern markets for specialty ingredients. Not only is it fun; you may expand your palate a bit too.

Tips for Shopping International Markets:

- Don't be afraid to ask questions.
- Show pictures for those lost-in-translation moments.
- Look at ingredient labels. Most are printed in English so you can spot any stabilizers, sugars, dyes, or unwanted ingredients.
- Explore the produce aisle! Most international markets will have things American supermarkets don't, like Korean melon, shiso or perilla leaves, lemongrass, or burdock root. Don't be afraid to buy some and experiment at home!

Things I Avoid

This book is not about restriction but about abundance on all levels to achieve effortless harmony. That said, there are items that I consistently steer away from, though I may still have them from time to time. I simply don't feel they help me thrive, and if anything, they can hinder my vitality, so I try to avoid these ingredients as much as I practically can:

- SOY PROTEIN (YOU'LL NOTICE THIS IS A PROTEIN-BASED RECIPE BOOK WITHOUT ANY TOFU)
- GMOS
- HYDROGENATED OILS
- CORN SYRUP
- CARRAGEENAN AND OTHER GUMS
- ARTIFICIAL FLAVORS OR COLORINGS
- PROCESSED FOODS
- IODIZED SALT
- WHITE FLOUR
- ENRICHED WHEAT
- WHITE SUGAR

On Sweets

The best part about this lifestyle is that there is always room for chocolate (it's neutral!). I strive for 65 percent cocoa or higher, but I've been known to go as low as 55 percent and am known to love a dark chocolate bar with sea salt and almonds. There are a few choice dessert recipes in the book to keep on hand for when the sweet tooth comes calling.

On Candida and Other Yeast

If you are experiencing issues with candida or other yeast, or are on certain types of medication, it's smart to stay away from sweet fruits, which can foster more yeast in your system. Instead, stick with low-sugar green juices of kale, celery, cucumber, fennel, romaine, lemon, and ginger.

On Oils

In his book *Become Younger*, Norman W. Walker writes, "When fats are raw, natural and uncooked as in avocado, olive oil, nuts, etc. and in nearly all vegetables in small quantities, the lymph nodes can emulsify them quickly and effectively, in which case they are promptly available for fuel and lubrication throughout the body. When the fats have been cooked, however, as in fried foods, the fat has been converted into an inorganic product . . . [which] results in the fat remaining in the circulation of the blood . . . clogging up the system instead of being available for constructive use." Does this mean we steer away from fat and oils altogether? No. Fat has important purposes in satiating us, imparting flavor and grounding us. But it is good to note that not all fats are created equal and it is helpful to be mindful about the type of fats we consume. This is why I cook mostly with avocado oil, which is easier to digest and, when cooking, has higher smoke points than cold-pressed oils like olive oil. I love olive oil but I use it mainly for salad dressings and drizzling after cooking. Coconut oil is great for cooking as well but imparts a coconut-y flavor, which works well for Southeast Asian and Indian-inspired dishes as well as baking, but not so much Italian or classic French.

A Note On Soy

Growing up half Asian, soy played a major role in my diet from soy sauce to tofu but it was used differently and more sparingly than the Western world. These days I avoid tofu and tempeh because it is highly processed and has been known to affect hormone levels if consumed for a long period of time. That's not to say I enjoy it from time to time and you'll see Tamari, which is a gluten-free soy sauce, is used liberally in the book. If you have a soy allergy, which many do, you can substitute tamari with coconut aminos or sea salt.

On Veganism

I am not a vegan, but my diet is mostly plant-based. I've learned from my experience with intuitive eating that subscribing to one specific way of eating does not serve me. It might, however, serve you. Whether it is for personal reasons, ethical reasons, environmental reasons—whatever your reasoning, it is not my business, nor is it anyone else's. Our society loves to label and categorize. Identifying as an intuitive eater confuses people and perhaps makes them uncomfortable because it holds a mirror up to their need to categorize themselves. I do believe living in a more plant-based way is the key to a higher-vibrating, more harmonious life.

On Portion Sizes

Doing away with the portions may be my favorite thing about food combining. I've never been a portion-controlling gal. Something in my soul craves abundance in all its forms, and this way of life opens up so much abundance. No more calorie counting, no more counting grams of . . . well . . . anything. Simply an abundance of plant-based whole foods. It's wonderfully freeing.

So, in keeping with that, the recommended servings in these recipes are really just suggestions. I've been known to house a family-size salad on the daily, or happily sip on thirty-two ounces of juice in the morning. The same applies to dinner. A little shift in perspective toward more salad, more dinner, in place of the portioned-out appetizer, main, and dessert.

Since restructuring the way I eat based on a few sets of food-combining rules, I've experienced stable weight loss, better skin, more energy, and just overall greater well-being.

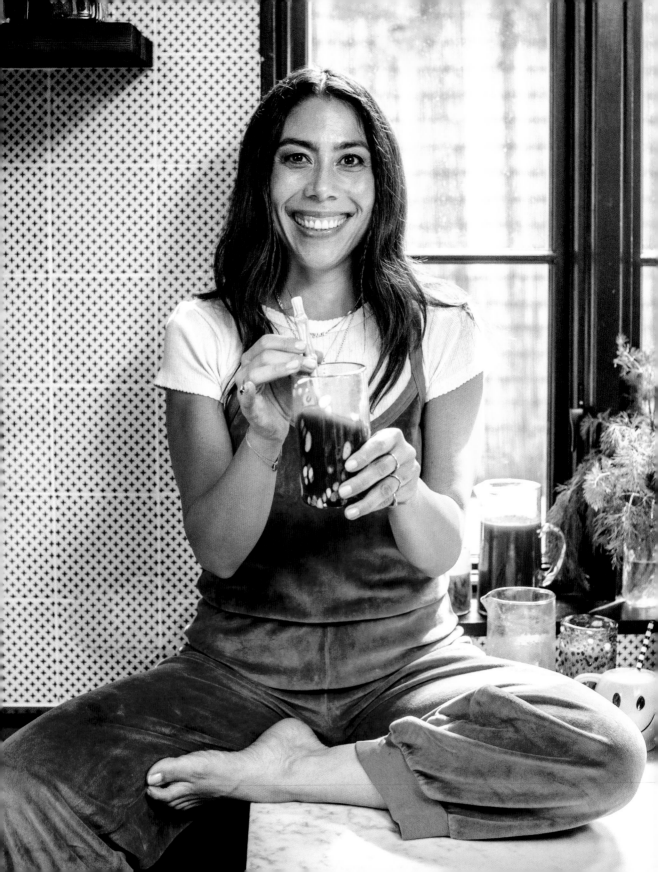

JUICES AND SMOOTHIES

GREEN LEMONADE

I call this the starter juice. The first green juice I ever had was made at the juice bar in the back of a health food shop in midtown Manhattan called Westerly Natural Market. I never knew green juice could taste so good, and it's what got me hooked for life. It's perfectly tart, slightly sweet, and you "can't taste the green," as they say. I could truly have this every day. In fact, I do, as does my whole family!

SERVES 1 TO 2 PEOPLE

INGREDIENTS

1 bunch (5 ounces/140 g) lacinato kale or dandelion greens

1 lemon, whole and unpeeled

2 green apples, quartered (15¾ ounces/450 g)

6 stalks celery (11 ounces/310 g)

Optional

3-inch (7.5-cm) knob ginger (2 ounces/55 g)

METHOD

Using a centrifugal juicer (if you have a masticating juicer, same quantities apply, you just might need to cut vegetables smaller), press all the ingredients through the feed chute. Enjoy juice immediately.

DRINK THE SUN

This is the most popular juice that we sell at Bonberi Mart, and it earns its name from the chlorophyll-rich goodness it is packed with. The most cleansing juice, and totally fruit-free, it is good if you are dealing with candida or other yeast issues, and it is still bright and delectable thanks to the lemon and ginger. You want the color of this to be a rich, almost opaque green. Remember, you can juice most fruits and vegetables whole, seeds, skin and all. The juicer does the work for you.

SERVES 1 TO 2 PEOPLE

INGREDIENTS

1 bunch (6¾ ounces/190 g) lacinato kale

5 to 7 stalks celery (9½ ounces/270 g)

1 large cucumber (7 ounces/200 g)

½ lemon

3-inch (7.5-cm) knob ginger (2 ounces/55 g) (see Note)

1 fennel bulb and stalks (22 ounces/343 g)

METHOD

Using an electric juicer, press all the ingredients through the feed chute. Enjoy the juice immediately.

Note: If you don't like your juice too gingery, go ahead and use less ginger than the recipe calls for.

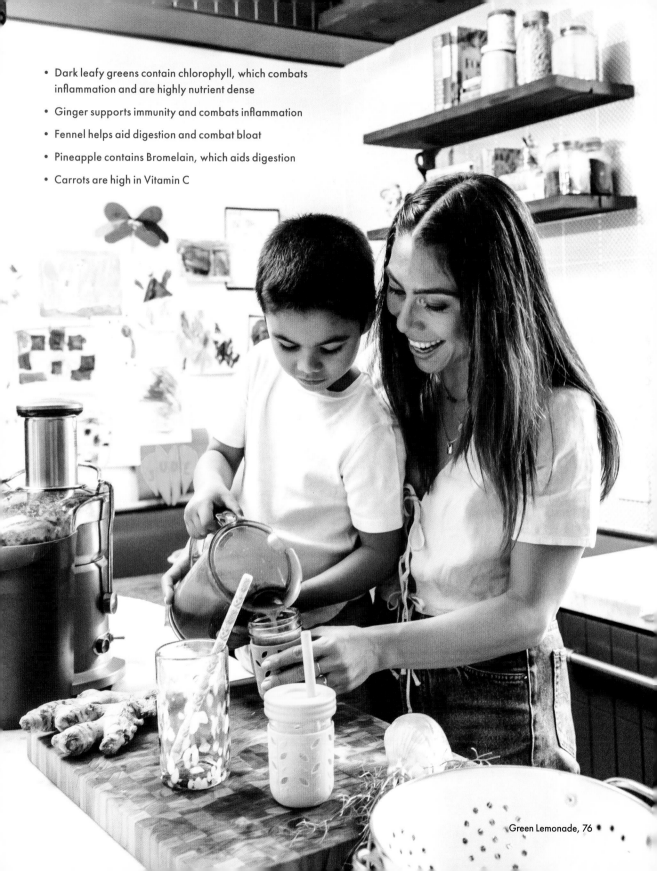

- Dark leafy greens contain chlorophyll, which combats inflammation and are highly nutrient dense
- Ginger supports immunity and combats inflammation
- Fennel helps aid digestion and combat bloat
- Pineapple contains Bromelain, which aids digestion
- Carrots are high in Vitamin C

Green Lemonade, 76

LA VIE EN ROUGE

Green juice usually gets all the buzz but root juices are incredibly healing and detoxifying too. Beet is known to boost energy, and what I love about this juice is it's fruit-free (so candida-friendly) yet naturally sweet thanks to the carrots and fennel. The ginger is anti-inflammatory and provides immune support while cutting through the sweetness perfectly. I include fennel and celery here to dilute the beet (both are incredibly anti-inflammatory), but you could totally use cucumber or romaine instead. If you're staying raw most of the day, I find this option to be an excellent mid-morning juice.

SERVES 1 TO 2 PEOPLE

INGREDIENTS

1 (1-pound/455-g) bag carrots

8 stalks celery

1 fennel bulb with stalks

2-inch (5-cm) knob ginger

½ large beet

Optional

1 pear (for a little more sweetness)

METHOD

Rinse all veggies and the pear, if using, and pat dry. Using an electric juicer, press all the ingredients through the feed chute. Enjoy the juice immediately.

TRUE BLOOD

I learned this recipe from my food combining teacher, Natalia Rose. The simplest recipe, this juice is slightly sweet from carrots yet candida-friendly. I call it True Blood, because it feels like an infusion of energy and life right into the blood. Plus, curiously, it tastes and looks like chocolate milk. You want basically a 1:1 ratio of carrot to romaine. I loved this juice when I was pregnant, and it's perfect if I'm getting over a stomach bug as it's nutrient packed and both very gentle and soothing to the tummy.

SERVES 1 TO 2 PEOPLE

INGREDIENTS

2 pounds (910 g) carrots

3 romaine hearts (23½ ounces/670 g)

METHOD

Rinse carrots and romaine hearts and pat dry. Using an electric juicer, press the carrots and romaine though the feed chute. Enjoy the juice immediately.

When using a centrifugal juicer, it's best to enjoy the juice right away. If using a slow-pressed juicer, the juice can last up to 3 days refrigerated.

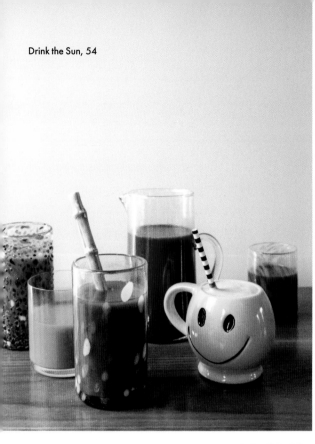
Drink the Sun, 54

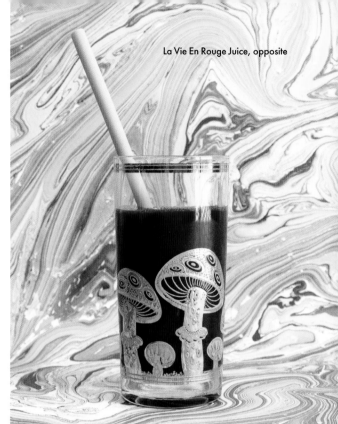
La Vie En Rouge Juice, opposite

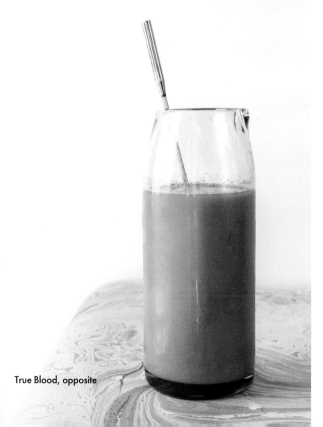
True Blood, opposite

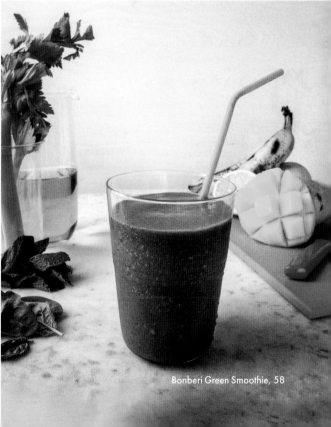
Bonberi Green Smoothie, 58

BONBERI GREEN SMOOTHIE

A lot of emphasis in the cleansing world is put on green juice—and rightfully so. It is the most healing plant food. But because it is so healing (read: detoxifying), if we are moving from a mainstream Western diet straight into juicing, the cleansing effects can sometimes lead to discomfort if we are not eliminating properly. One way to ease ourselves into the cleansing life without the side effects is the green smoothie. Packed with all the alkalinity, anti-inflammatory benefit, and hydration of green juice, it also maintains the ingredients' fiber and helps scrub the body of old waste, which requires some digestion and allows for a slower breakdown than a juice. A blended salad, if you will.

Here's the thing about this smoothie, though, which makes it different from other smoothies. It is properly food combined, so since it has fruit, there are no nuts, seeds, seed butters, protein powders, or any of the other junk—yes, I said junk—often thrown into a smoothie. I'm not sure when smoothies became dumping grounds for everything but the kitchen sink, but when you start getting complicated with your smoothie, you are no longer talking about a cleansing agent. It's just something to keep you full. The concept of cleansing smoothies is that they gently help elimination while giving you sustained energy. You could swap in other fruits here—replace the mango with pear, apple, orange, pineapple, or papaya—but I find this exact combo to be foolproof in flavor. If you are craving something even more satiating, you could add half an avocado, which is technically a fruit.

SERVES 1 TO 2 PEOPLE

INGREDIENTS

1 cup (140 g) frozen mango cubes

2 stalks celery, roughly chopped

Juice ½ lemon

1 handful or ⅓ cup (10 g) packed mint leaves

2 cups (60 g) packed baby spinach

1 frozen ripe banana, cut into 1-inch slices

2–3 cups (480–720 ml) raw coconut water (I like Copra or Harmless Harvest) or filtered water

METHOD

In a blender or food processor, blend all the ingredients. Enjoy! The smoothie can be stored in the fridge for 24 hours.

COCONUT SMOOTHIE

Back in the day, the original Liquiteria on Second Avenue was the place to be. They made the most amazing fresh juices and smoothies. This was a concoction I made up as a custom order there, when I first started the cleansing life, as a heartier drink during summer afternoons when I still wanted to keep raw. It tastes like a milkshake and is divine.

Tip: Wait until your bananas are spotted and ripe. This is when they are at their sweetest and best able to promote elimination. I also like to slice my bananas and then freeze them in advance to make for quick smoothies in the morning.

SERVES 1 TO 2 PEOPLE

INGREDIENTS

1 cup (240 g) frozen young coconut, defrosted

1 cup (210 g) frozen ripe banana, cut into 1-inch slices

1 cup (250 ml) raw coconut water

Dash of cinnamon

METHOD

In a blender or food processor, blend all the ingredients until creamy. Enjoy the smoothie immediately.

LUCKY SEVEN SHAKE

Not just for Saint Paddy's Day, this mint chip-y shake tastes exactly like ice cream and is refreshing all year round.

SERVES 1 TO 2 PEOPLE

INGREDIENTS

2 frozen ripe bananas, cut into 1-inch slices

1 to 2 dates, pitted (see Note)

1¾ cups (420 ml) almond milk, unsweetened

2 cups (60 g) packed baby spinach

½ teaspoon chlorella or spirulina

½ teaspoon mint extract

Dash of salt

2 tablespoons cacao nibs (1 tablespoon for garnish)

Garnish

Mint leaves

METHOD

In a blender or food processor, blend the bananas, dates, milk, spinach, chlorella, mint extract, salt, and 1 tablespoon of the cacao nibs until creamy. Garnish with 1 tablespoon of the cacao nibs and the mint leaves. Serve the smoothie immediately.

Note: Whether to use 1 or 2 dates depends on how sweet you like your shake.

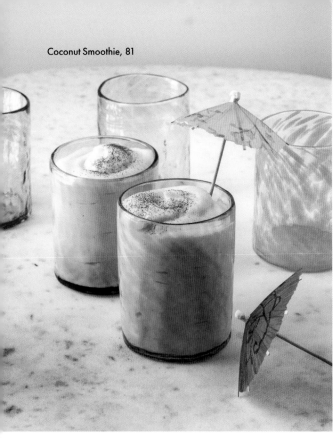
Coconut Smoothie, 81

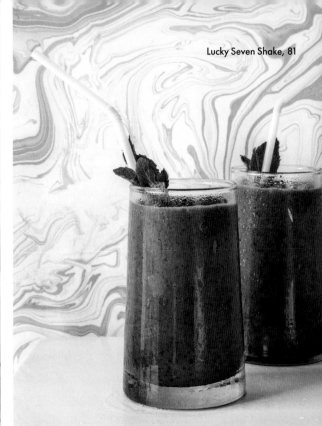
Lucky Seven Shake, 81

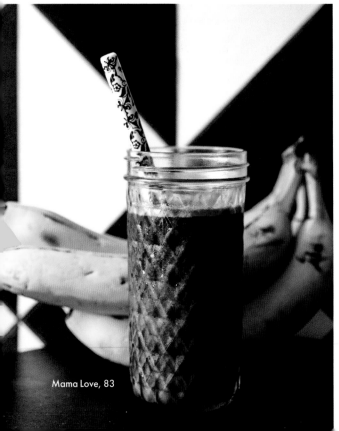
Mama Love, 83

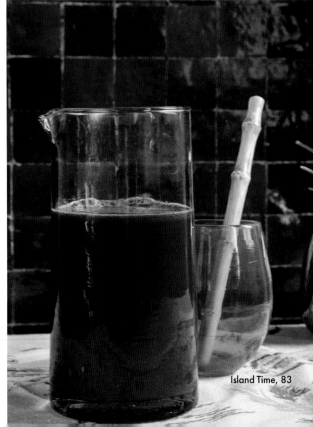
Island Time, 83

MAMA LOVE

I created this recipe when I was pregnant and would order a similar one at the now-shuttered Integral Yoga Natural Foods, a dusty little hippy joint in the West Village that made the best juices and smoothies. It is packed with chlorophyll from the spirulina and spinach, is dense and filling from the almond butter, and is omega-rich from the flax seeds, and it also has dates for softening the cervix. This smoothie is a slight-food combine bend with the almond butter and bananas, but when you're looking for something heartier, it's a good option. This is truly a superfood smoothie, whether you are expecting or nursing or neither!

SERVES 1 TO 2 PEOPLE

INGREDIENTS

2 frozen ripe bananas, cut into 1-inch slices

1 cup (30 g) packed baby spinach

2 tablespoons raw almond butter

1 date, pitted

1 teaspoon spirulina powder or granules

1½ cups (360 ml) water (see Note)

½ teaspoon ground cinnamon

Optional

1 tablespoon ground flax seeds

METHOD

In a blender or food processor, blend all the ingredients. Enjoy the smoothie immediately.

Note: You can substitute 1 to 2 cups unsweetened almond milk for the water. One cup milk will make a smoothie with the consistency of ice cream, and 2 cups a thinner one.

ISLAND TIME

I make this juice a few days a week. It's slightly sweet but tart thanks to the cilantro. (You can sub other herbs if you're not a fan.) Pineapple is packed with bromelain, which is a group of digestive enzymes that combats indigestion and bloating. Plus, this fruit adds a hint of the tropics, which makes me feel like I'm on vacation.

SERVES 1 TO 2 PEOPLE

INGREDIENTS

1 bunch (6¾ ounces/190 g) lacinato kale

5 to 7 stalks celery (9½ ounces/270 g)

1 lime, whole and unpeeled

3-inch (7.5-cm) knob ginger (2 ounces/55 g)

1 bunch cilantro

2 cups (330 g) peeled, cored, and speared pineapple

METHOD

Rinse vegetables and pat dry. Using an electric juicer, press all the ingredients through the feed chute. Serve the juice immediately.

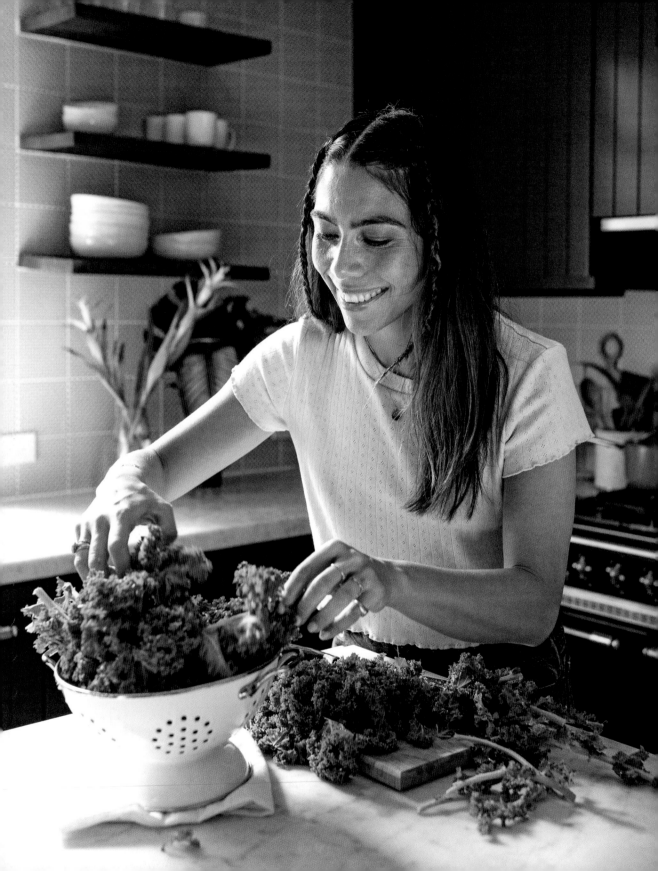

SALADS

DULSE CAESAR SALAD

Caesar salad might unequivocally be the perfect salad. Cold, crisp romaine dripping with tangy, garlicky dressing with a dusting of cheesy and peppery goodness. I could never really vibe with the health food versions—piled-high kale topped with toasted nori and some kind of hemp cheese situation. The one I prefer is not shrouded in hippy regalia. I'm talking about the earnest version you get at a steakhouse, where they ceremoniously arrive at your table wielding a gigantic wooden bowl and proceed to rub the entire thing with garlic before dumping the salad in (a trick my dad taught me before I was ten). What really makes this is the dulse, a briny algae that's, yes, packed with trace minerals and antioxidants, but also is a solid dupe for anchovies. If you can't find dulse, nori or seaweed will work fine. Just don't go easy on the pepper—"twist," as my dad would say, "until your arm gets tired." Because this salad is neutral, you can top it with avocado, a grain, or grilled protein. You could even make the dressing and use it as a dip for crudités. It happily goes with everything!

SERVES 2

INGREDIENTS

2 heads romaine

½ cup (120 ml) Dulse Caesar Dressing (page 214)

Garnish

1 teaspoon nutritional yeast

1 teaspoon chopped fresh parsley leaves

Freshly cracked black pepper

METHOD

Rinse the romaine and pat dry with paper towels. Wrap the leaves in a dish towel and refrigerate until ready to use; you want them to be ice-cold and crisp. Once the dressing is made, roughly chop the chilled lettuce; I like 1-inch (2.5-cm) bite-size pieces. Place the romaine in a large salad bowl. Pour the dressing over the leaves and toss with tongs until well coated. Sprinkle with the yeast and parsley and toss again. Generously crack the pepper over the salad. Serve immediately.

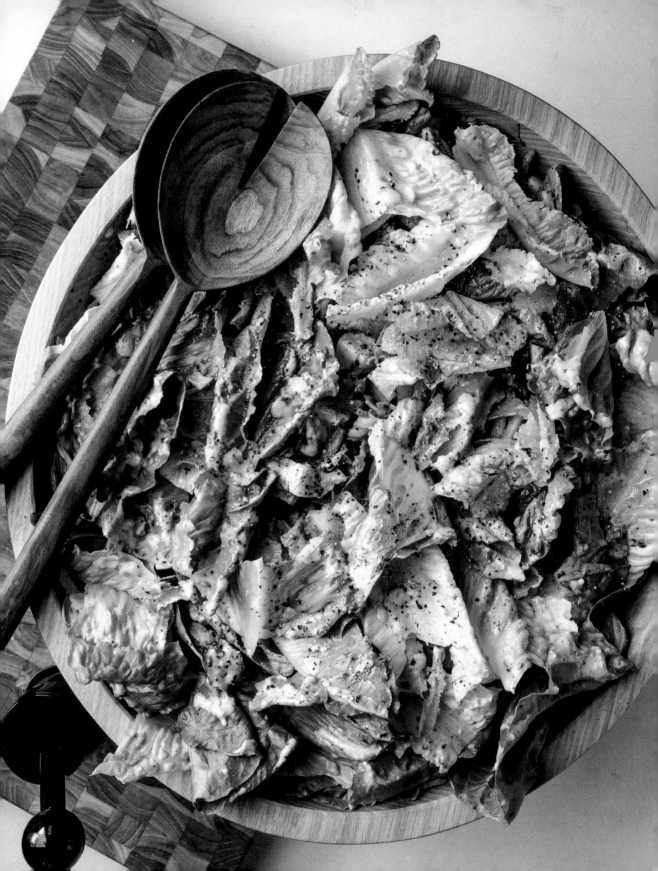

NORI SALAD WRAPS

One of the first food combining principles that really stuck with me is having a raw salad before any cooked meal. Raw vegetables contain live enzymes that help the body digest food. Consider them your alkaline armor for the meal to come. The thing is, sometimes it's a drag to make and eat a salad (yeah, I said it). This recipe combines my Korean-DNA wrapping of just about everything in seaweed with the foundational food combining principle of eating light to heavy to ensure energy and vitality. You can really get creative here and add any raw veg you like—shaved fennel, sprouts, kale, cabbage, the list goes on. The idea is to pack the wrap with a ton of fresh veg with a savory schmear, then roll and dip! Because what's more fun than a roll?

MAKES 4 WRAPS

INGREDIENTS

4 raw or toasted sheets nori

4 teaspoons Beet Gochujang (page 235)

4 leaves Boston lettuce, red or green leaf

1 firm but ripe avocado, sliced

1 large handful sprouts, or pea shoots (I love pea shoots, broccoli sprouts, or microgreens)

2 Persian cucumbers, thinly sliced

2 carrots, shaved

2 radishes, thinly sliced

Small bowl of room-temperature water

For serving

Tamari sauce

Dash of sesame seeds

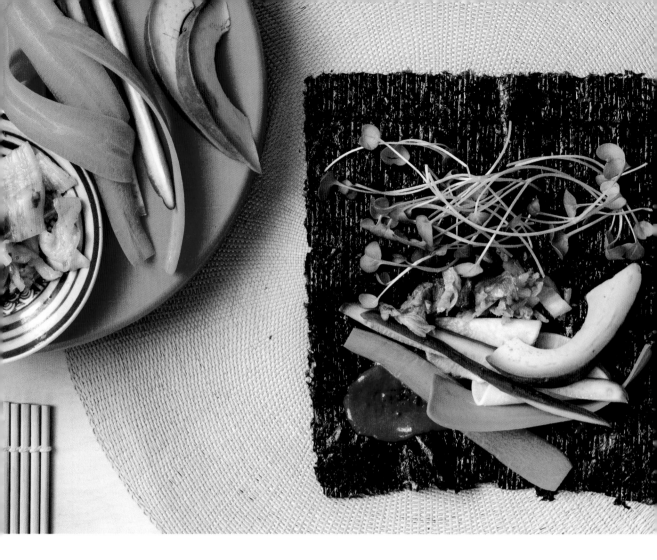

METHOD

Along the bottom edge of each sheet of nori, spread 1 teaspoon of the gochujang. Then place 1 leaf lettuce on top of the paste. Next, arrange the sliced avocado, sprouts, cucumbers, carrots, and radishes (or whatever veggies you are subbing) in a row, on top of the lettuce. You don't want the roll to be too large, or it will be hard to seal. Using both hands, gently tuck the bottom edge of the nori and roll to the top. Dip your finger in the water to wet the top edge, and seal the roll. Slice diagonally with a sharp knife. Serve with tamari sauce topped with a dash of sesame seeds for dipping!

I like to have these wraps before dinner instead of a salad. For a group, serve all the ingredients in small bowls to make a fun DIY bar.

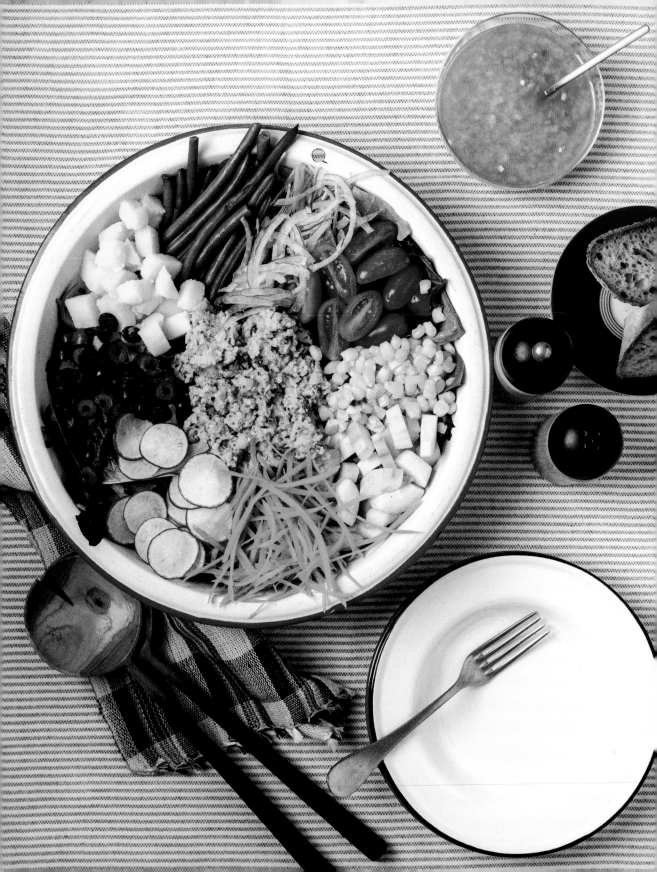

CHICKPEA NIÇOISE

When I was fifteen, I spent the summer in Nice. I lived in a former convent on a cliff overlooking the ocean and would study films starring Jean Reno, learn popular French songs, go to tiny subterranean discotheques on the weekend, and at lunch descend to the convent cafeteria and eat hot baguettes, every day. It was heaven. This is where I discovered my favorite food. Salade Niçoise. I could not get enough of it. My classmates would make fun of me because I would order it at every meal, at every brasserie and bistro that had it on the menu (and they all did.) The salty olives, the juicy boiled potatoes, the perfectly crisp haricots verts—it was the perfect dish.

SERVES 4 TO 6

INGREDIENTS

1 large russet potato, peeled and cut into ½-inch (2.5-cm) cubes

1 teaspoon sea salt

2 cups (225 g) haricot verts, ends trimmed

2 cups (480 ml) ice water

1 cup (175 g) Chickpea Tuna (page 142)

1 cup (150 g) frozen corn kernels, thawed

1 cup (105 g) pitted black, kalamata, or Niçoise olives, sliced ½ large cucumber, peeled, seeded, and sliced

¼ red onion, thinly sliced

1 cup (150 g) grape or cherry tomatoes, halved

2 carrots, grated on a large box cutter

½ cup (55 g) radishes, thinly sliced

4 cups (140 g) mixed greens

2 Belgian endives, thinly sliced

1 cup (240 ml) Bistro Shallot Vinaigrette (page 212)

METHOD

In a small pot, combine the potato with 4 cups (960 ml) water and ½ teaspoon of the salt. Bring to a boil, and boil the potato until tender, about 5 minutes. Drain and let cool; set aside.

In a shallow pan, combine the haricots verts with 3 cups (720 ml) water and ½ teaspoon of the salt. Bring to a boil and blanch the haricots verts, 3 to 5 minutes. Drain and submerge in 2 cups (480 ml) ice water to prevent cooking. After a few minutes, drain and set aside.

In a large serving bowl, combine the greens and endives. Add the chickpea tuna, corn, olives, potato, haricots verts, cucumber, onion, tomatoes, carrots, and radishes in a circle over the greens and endives. Pour over the dressing and serve.

MASSAGED KALE WITH CURRANTS AND SUNFLOWER SEEDS

There was a little English meat-pie vendor in Chelsea Market years back. Yes, you heard that right, meat pies. But they served the most glorious vegan kale salad. Heaps of fluffy shaved kale with a light, creamy tahini dressing punctuated by sunflower seeds and dried currants. Just the perfect salad. This is my homage.

SERVES 2 TO 4

INGREDIENTS

1 bunch curly kale

½ cup (120 ml) Liquid Gold Dressing (page 216)

½ cup (55 g) dried currants

¼ cup (35 g) raw sunflower seeds

2 scallions, sliced

½ cup (75 g) sliced radish

Flaky sea salt

Freshly cracked black pepper

METHOD

Pull the kale leaves off the stems (save the stems for juicing), and in a large bowl, tear the leaves into bite-size pieces. For a finer chopped salad, pulse leaves in a food processor or blender for a few seconds and transfer to bowl. Pour the dressing over the kale and massage well with your hands. Add the currants, sunflower seeds, scallions, and radish. Add salt and pepper to taste and serve in individual bowls.

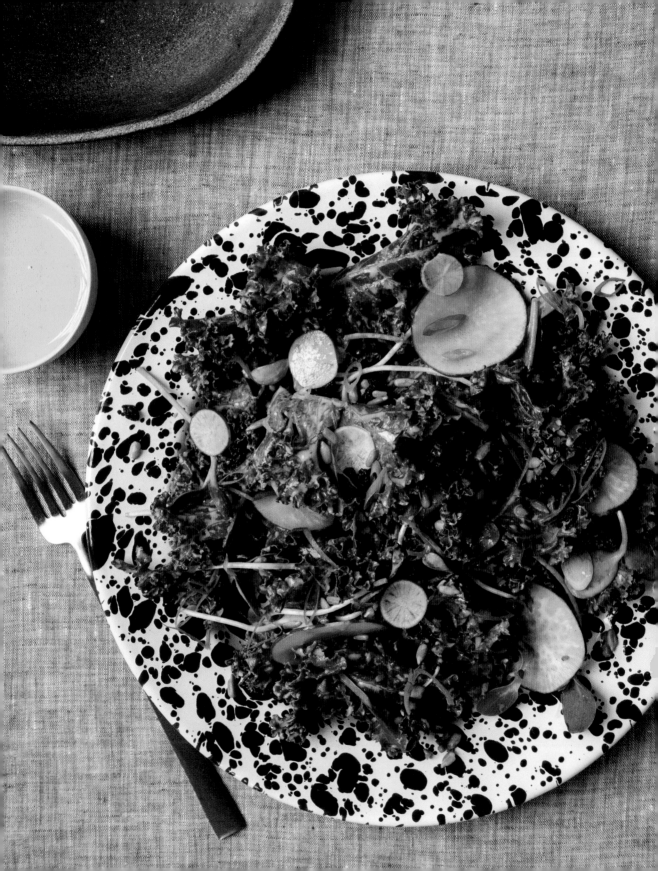

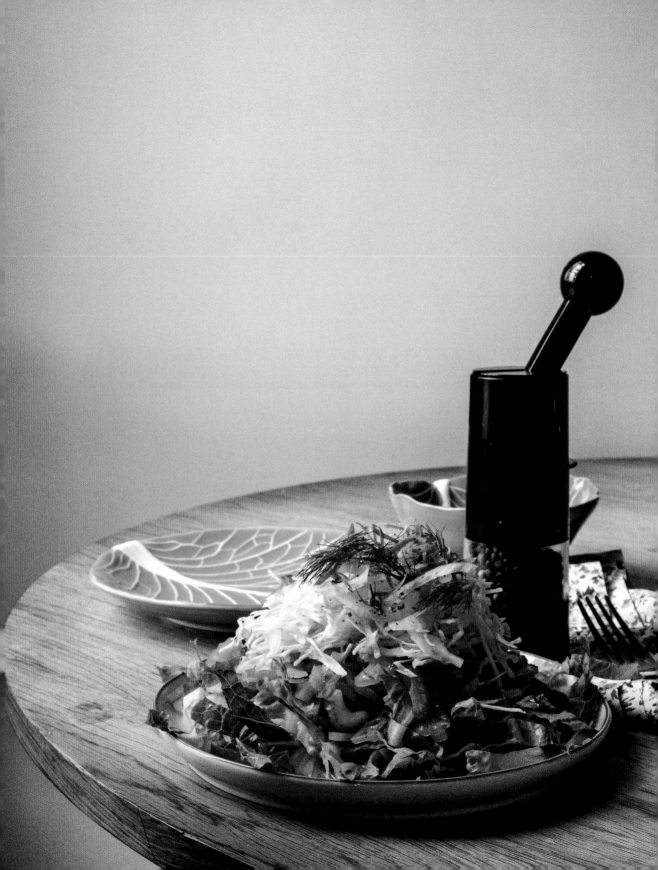

MAROULI SALAD

At Greek restaurants, *horiatiki*, or village salads, usually get all the glory. And why shouldn't they, they're perfect. But this little-known salad is a sleeper hit. I usually order it with my meal since it's the perfect combination of crunchy hydrating romaine, bright herbs, and tangy dressing. It goes with everything!

SERVES 2 TO 4

INGREDIENTS

For the salad

3 heads romaine

2 cups (160 g) shaved white cabbage, thinly sliced

1 cup (85 g) very thinly sliced white onion

2 stalks celery, thinly sliced

2 scallions, thinly sliced

For the dressing

MAKES ¾ CUP (180 ML) DRESSING

½ cup (235 ml) olive oil

Juice of 2 lemons

1 clove garlic, grated

1 teaspoon sea salt

Cracked black pepper

2 tablespoons chopped fresh dill

2 tablespoons capers

METHOD

Make the salad: Rinse the romaine and pat dry with paper towels. (If needed, wrap the leaves in a dish towel and place in the fridge to keep them crisp.) In a large bowl, combine the romaine with the cabbage, onion, celery, and scallions and set aside.

Make the dressing: In a small bowl, combine all the dressing ingredients and whisk until emulsified. Pour the dressing over the salad and toss. Serve immediately.

MEXICAN CHOP

This salad is an homage to the taco salads I'd get as a kid in those massive tortilla bowls. Packed with veggies, tossed with a slightly creamy, sweet vinaigrette and finished with some obligatory crunch.

SERVES 2 TO 4

INGREDIENTS

2 small heads romaine, very thinly sliced

4 large carrots, chopped

1 cup (80 g) chopped yellow, green, or red bell pepper

1 avocado, chopped

½ red onion, chopped

1 jalapeño chile, seeded and chopped

¼ cup (4 g) chopped cilantro leaves

1 cup (240 g/8 ounces) canned garbanzo beans, drained and rinsed

¾ cup (180 ml) Honey Lime Vinaigrette (at right)

Optional

1 cup (31 g) crushed tortilla chips

METHOD

In a large bowl, combine the romaine, carrots, pepper, avocado, onion, jalapeño, cilantro, and beans. Pour the dressing over the salad and toss. Crumble chips on top, if using, and serve.

HONEY LIME VINAIGRETTE

I consider this the perfect summer salad dressing, but you could have it year-round. The tartness of the lime married with the sweetness of the honey (or maple syrup, if you're vegan) tastes like backyard BBQs and long, hot pool days.

MAKES 1 CUP (240 ML) DRESSING

INGREDIENTS

½ teaspoon ground cumin

2 tablespoons raw honey or maple syrup

1 clove garlic, grated

Dash of cayenne pepper

½ cup (120 ml) Aquafaba Mayo (page 223) or store-bought vegan mayo

½ teaspoon sea salt

¼ cup (60 ml) olive oil

2 tablespoons apple cider vinegar

Juice of 1 lime

METHOD

In a bowl, whisk all the ingredients, or blend in a food processor until creamy. Store the dressing in the fridge in an airtight container for up to a week.

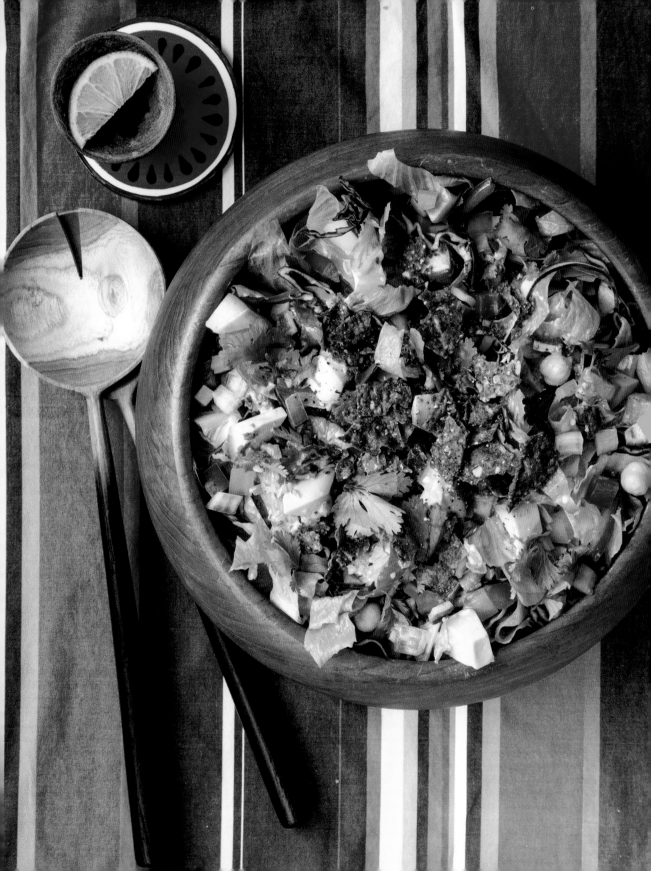

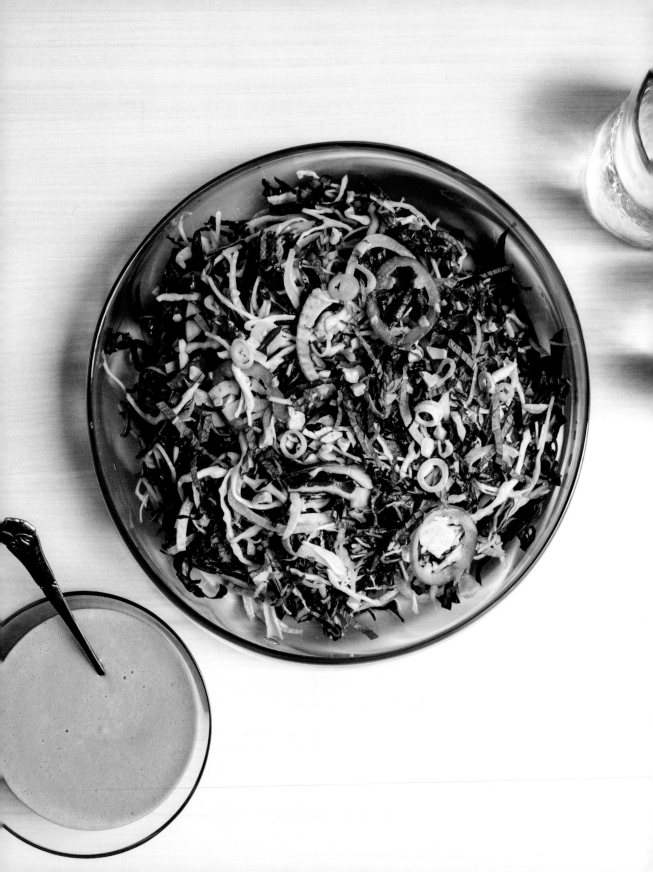

CRUNCHY PEANUT KALE SALAD

Kale salad. Groundbreaking. But, honestly, this version kind of is. The mix of shaved cabbage and fennel gives this chlorophyll-packed dish the crunch it deserves, with an earthy salty-sweet dressing you could drink. I could have this salad every day.

SERVES 2 TO 4

INGREDIENTS

2 bunches (11¾ ounces/335 g) lacinato kale, thinly sliced

1 fennel bulb (10 ounces/280 g), thinly sliced

1 cup (90 g) shaved and very thinly sliced white cabbage

½ red onion (6¼ ounces/175 g), thinly sliced

1 bunch mint

2 scallions, thinly sliced

1 jalapeño chile, seeded and thinly sliced

½ cup (85 g) roughly chopped peanuts

½ cup (120 ml) Peanut Ginger Dressing (page 220)

METHOD

In a large bowl, combine the kale, fennel, cabbage, onion, mint, scallions, jalapeño, and peanuts. Pour the dressing over the salad and toss, coating all the ingredients well. Serve. The salad will keep in the fridge for up to 2 days.

SIMPLE MASSAGED KALE SALAD WITH BEETS AND AVOCADO

The simplicity of this salad makes it a dish that I'll turn to again and again. It's my favorite of the salads that we sell at Bonberi Mart for this reason. The combination of fluffy kale, broken down by massaging in a tangy vinaigrette, with grounding quinoa is the height of satisfaction for me. You can omit the quinoa to keep the salad neutral.

SERVES 2 TO 4

INGREDIENTS

2 medium beets, peeled and chopped

1 bunch curly kale

1 watermelon radish, thinly sliced

1 avocado, cubed into ½-inch cubes

Optional

2 cups (220 g) cooked quinoa

½ cup (120 ml) Basic Vinaigrette with 1 tablespoon of maple syrup (page 212)

METHOD

Fill a pot with 3 inches (7.5 cm) of water. Place the beets in a steamer basket inside the pot and bring to a boil. Reduce to a simmer. Cover the pot and steam the beets for 25 to 30 minutes, until tender.

Cook the quinoa as directed on packaging, if using, and let cool.

While the beets are steaming, pull the kale leaves off the stems (you'll need about 5 cups/ 190 g, packed), tear the leaves into bite-size pieces, and place in a large bowl. (Save the stems for juicing.)

In a large bowl, combine the beets, quinoa, and kale and add the radish, and avocado. Pour the dressing over the salad and toss. Serve immediately or store in the fridge for up to 2 days.

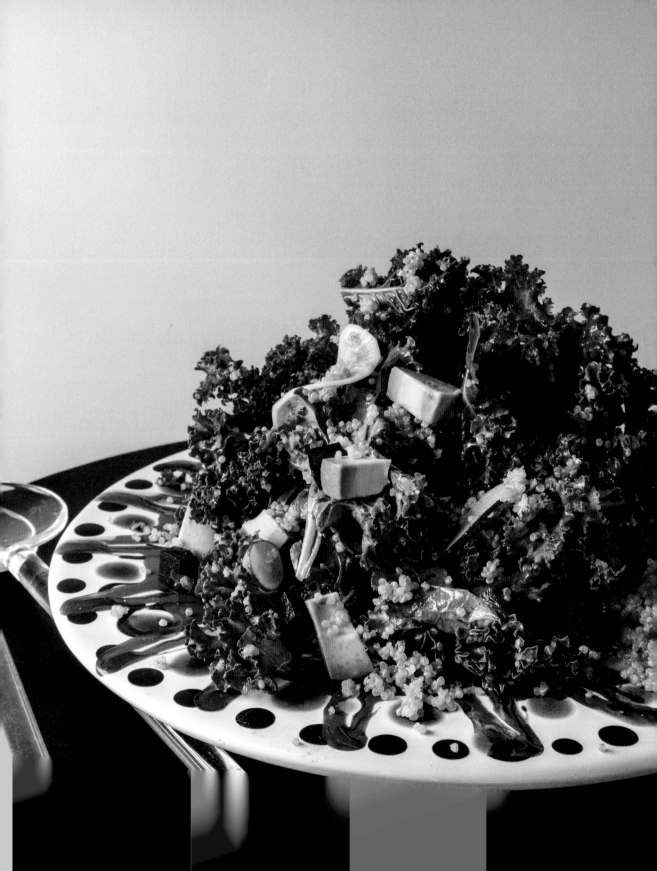

ITALIAN CHOPPED SALAD

This reminds me of the kind of salad you'd get at a power lunch—people still power lunch, don't they? Served on a fancy white plate in a fancy restaurant uptown, it has everything you want: bitter greens, briny olives, sweet peas, and hearty herbed beans, it's super filling and delicious. At home you can serve it however you want.

SERVES 4

INGREDIENTS

2 cups (40 g) arugula

½ cup (140 g) shaved fennel

1 cup (40 g) thinly sliced radicchio

2 radishes, thinly sliced

1 bell pepper, thinly sliced

½ cup (150 g) grape tomatoes, halved

½ cup (65 g) pitted Castelvetrano olives

4 sun-dried tomatoes, hydrated and chopped

1 cup (135 g) frozen sweet peas, thawed

1 cup (155 g) Herby Garbanzo Beans (recipe follows)

½ cup (120 ml) Italian House Dressing (page 215)

HERBY GARBANZO BEANS

MAKES 1 CUP

INGREDIENTS

1 cup (240 g/8 ounces) canned garbanzo beans, drained and rinsed

½ teaspoon dried thyme

1 clove garlic, grated

Juice of ½ lemon

1 tablespoon olive oil

Sea salt

Freshly cracked black pepper

METHOD

Make the salad: In a large bowl, combine the arugula, fennel, radicchio, radishes, bell pepper, grape tomatoes, olives, sun-dried tomatoes, and peas.

Make the herby garbanzo beans: In a bowl, combine the beans, thyme, garlic, lemon juice, and oil, and salt and pepper to taste.

Top the salad with the beans. Pour the dressing over the salad. Toss and serve.

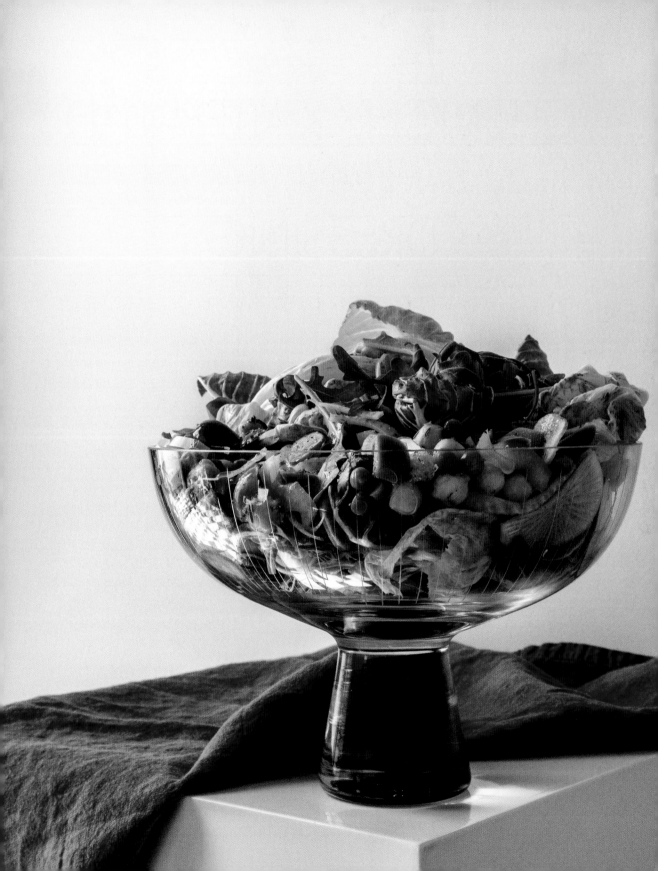

CRUNCHY KALE SALAD WITH UNIVERSAL DRESSING

ore kale. But it's the dressing that makes this one. If you've been following along, you know that the secret to a solid kale salad is the crunch. No one wants a gloppy mess, especially if you're going with a creamy dressing. And this salad hits all the points.

SERVES 2 TO 4

INGREDIENTS

1 bunch (6¾ ounces/190 g) kale

1 large cucumber (11¾ ounces/335 g), peeled and seeded

4 stalks celery, chopped

2 scallions, chopped

1 fennel bulb (10 ounces/280 g), thinly sliced

½ cup (120 ml) Tahini Green Goddess Dressing (page 221)

METHOD

Pull the kale leaves from the stems and tear the leaves into bite-size pieces. (You'll need about 1 packed cup/65 grams. Save the stems for juicing.) In a large serving bowl, combine the kale, cucumber, celery, scallions, and fennel. Drizzle with the dressing and toss to evenly coat the kale with the creamy dressing. Serve.

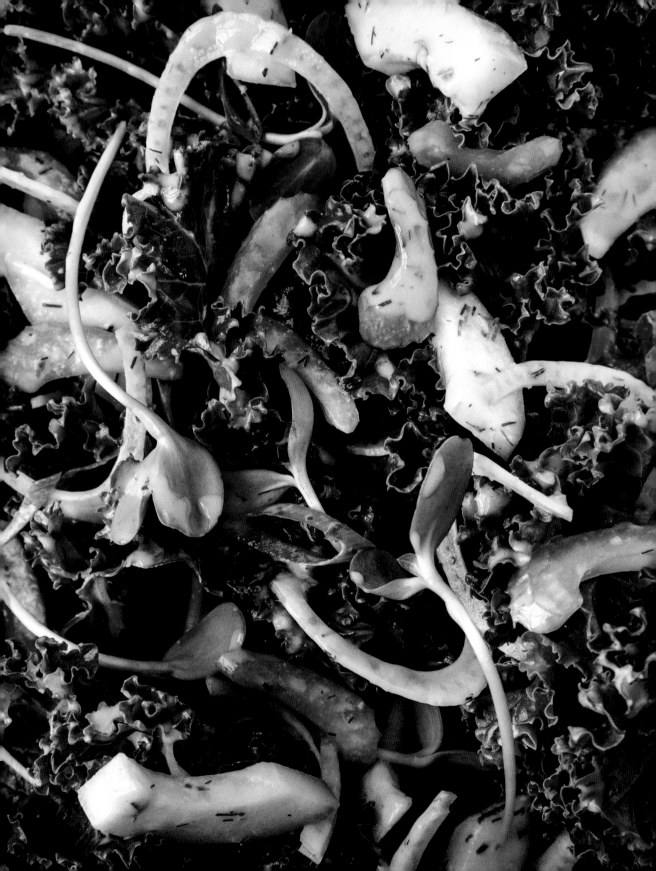

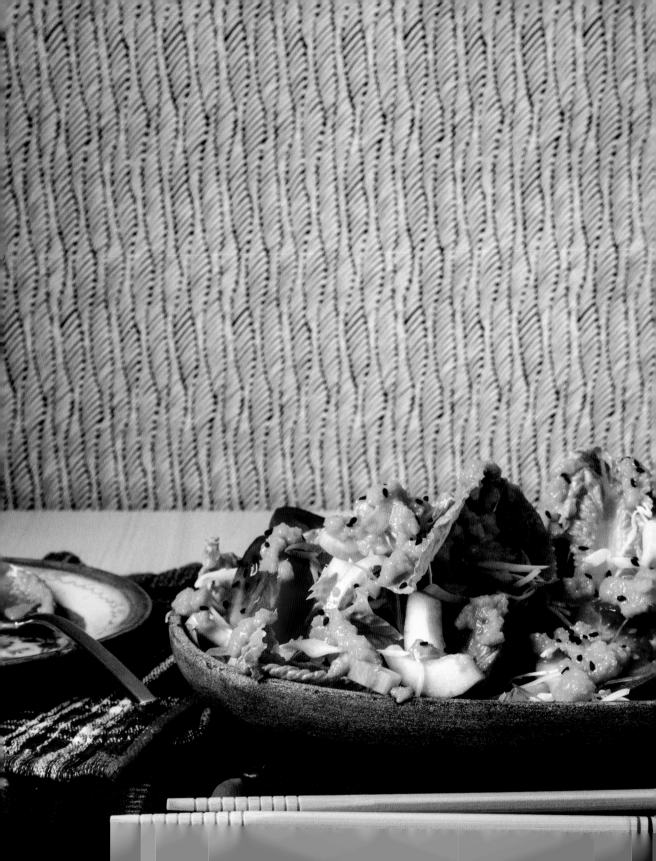

JAPANESE HOUSE SALAD

This salad is a nod to that quintessential carrot-ginger dressed salad you get at local sushi joints that usually involves a hunk of iceberg lettuce, a hefty wedge of tomato, and some cucumber rounds for good measure. It's wonderfully ubiquitous but nearly impossible to get right—until now.

SERVES 2 TO 4

INGREDIENTS

2 heads (1 pound/455 g) romaine, roughly chopped

½ cup (40 g) white cabbage, thinly sliced

1 large cucumber, peeled and seeded

1 large tomato, sliced into thick wedges

¼ white onion, thinly sliced

½ cup (120 ml) Japanese House (page 216)

Garnish

1 tablespoon sesame seeds or gomasio

1 scallion, chopped

METHOD

In a large serving bowl, combine the romaine, cabbage, cucumber, tomato, and onion. Pour the dressing over the salad. Garnish with sesame seeds and scallion. Serve immediately.

PICNIC COLE SLAW

This might be an unpopular opinion, but I love cole slaw. I love the super creamy kinds and I love the lighter types—I don't discriminate. I do understand the aversion to the traditional mushy variety that's given slaw its bad name. This version has an Asian spin but it's versatile, to go with anything from your backyard BBQ to your own pre-dinner.

SERVES 4 TO 6

INGREDIENTS

4 cups (325 g) thinly sliced or shredded white cabbage

2 cups (155 g) thinly sliced or shredded red cabbage

4 medium carrots, peeled and thinly sliced

4 scallions, minced

1 bunch chives, minced

¼ cup (18 g) fresh cilantro, roughly chopped

For the dressing

½ cup (120 ml) Aquafaba Mayo (page 223) or your favorite vegan mayo (see Note)

2 teaspoons rice vinegar or apple cider vinegar

½ teaspoon sea salt

Freshly cracked black pepper

2 teaspoons toasted sesame oil

1 teaspoon coconut sugar

Optional

¼ cup (25 g) roasted peanuts, roughly chopped

METHOD

In a large bowl, combine the white and red cabbage, carrots, scallions, chives, and cilantro. In a medium bowl, whisk together all the dressing ingredients until well blended. Pour over the cabbage mixture. Massage well with your hands. Top with peanuts, if using, for an extra crunch. Serve immediately or store in an airtight container for up to 3 days.

Note: You can add more mayo if you'd like a creamier consistency.

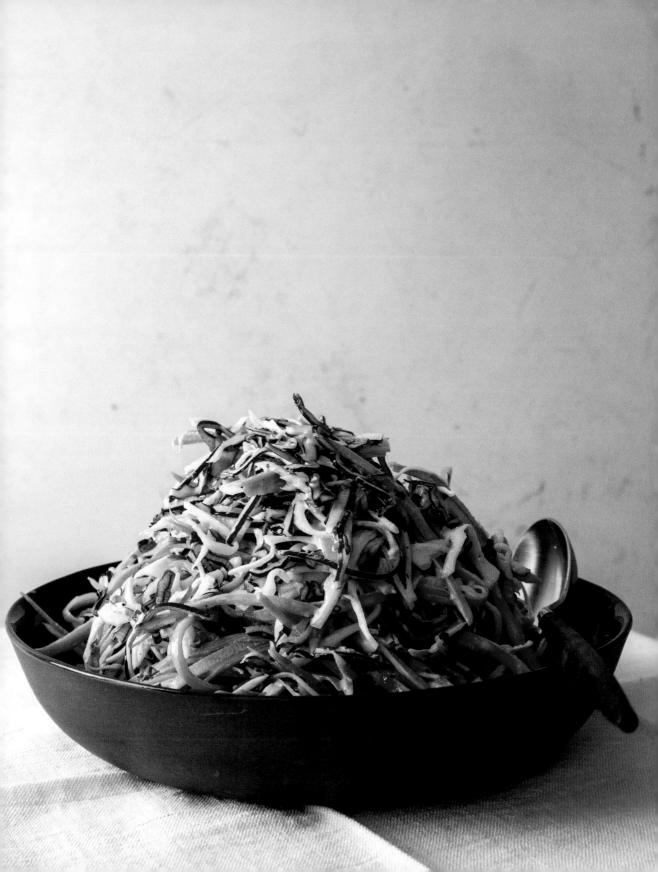

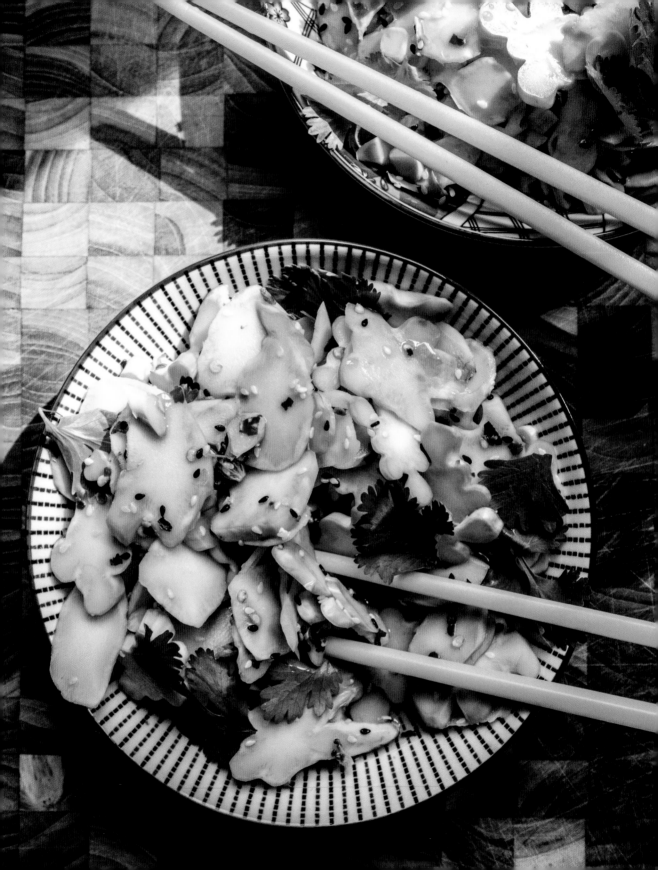

QUICK PICKLED BROCCOLI STEM SALAD

The town I grew up in has a famous joint called Baumgart's Cafe, which was part retro American diner, part Chinese restaurant. They are known for their ice cream sodas, burgers and fries—and dumplings. With the dumplings came this tangy broccoli stem salad that was so incredibly tart, so incredibly crunchy and garlicky, that I've always wanted to re-create it. They've since taken it off the menu, so here is your only chance.

SERVES 1 TO 2

INGREDIENTS

Stems from 2 to 3 heads broccoli, or 1 to 2 cups (150 g to 300 g) sliced broccoli stems

½ cup (120 ml) white rice vinegar

½ cup (120 ml) filtered water

1 teaspoon sea salt

2 tablespoons coconut sugar

1 teaspoon grated ginger

2 to 3 cloves garlic, minced

Optional

1 teaspoon toasted sesame oil

Chili flakes

Black sesame seeds

Fresh cilantro leaves

Flaky sea salt

METHOD

Peel the rough outer layer of the broccoli stems using a vegetable peeler or paring knife. Thinly slice the peeled stems on a diagonal. You don't want them paper thin, but they shouldn't be too thick either. Set aside. In a medium bowl, whisk together the vinegar, water, salt, sugar, ginger, and garlic. Add the broccoli stems and let sit in marinade to pickle for 30 minutes or overnight.

Drain the stems. Drizzle with the oil and top with the chili flakes, sesame seeds, cilantro, and salt, if using. Serve. You can let the stems sit in the pickling solution in an airtight container for up to a week.

JOE'S CHOPPED SALAD

T his salad is an homage to Joe's Stone Crab. Every New Year's Eve, my family stops by the Miami institution to pick up dinner to go and I always opt for this massive chopped salad. The original has eggs, peanuts, and feta, which I omit because the real magic is in the chunky, tangy dressing.

SERVES 2 TO 4

INGREDIENTS

1 head organic iceberg, or 2 hearts romaine (1½ pounds/680 g total)

1 large cucumber, chopped and seeded

1 large tomato

2 large carrots, peeled and chopped

1 cup (115 g) pitted black olives, sliced

½ red onion, thinly sliced

1 cup (240 g/8 ounces) canned garbanzo beans, drained and rinsed

1 cup (240ml) Joe's Chop Dressing (recipe follows)

Optional

¼ cup (85 g) feta or vegan feta

JOE'S CHOP DRESSING

MAKES 1½ CUPS

INGREDIENTS

½ cup (120 ml) olive oil

¼ cup (60 ml) apple cider vinegar

2 tablespoons maple syrup

2 tablespoons parsley

1 shallot, minced

2 tablespoons capers

½ cup (120 ml) water

Dash of cayenne pepper

½ teaspoon sea salt

Freshly cracked black pepper

METHOD

In a large bowl, combine the iceberg, cucumber, tomato, carrots, olives, onion, and beans—plus the feta, if using. In a small bowl, whisk all the dressing ingredients together. You want the dressing to be very chunky. Pour it over the salad and toss. Serve immediately.

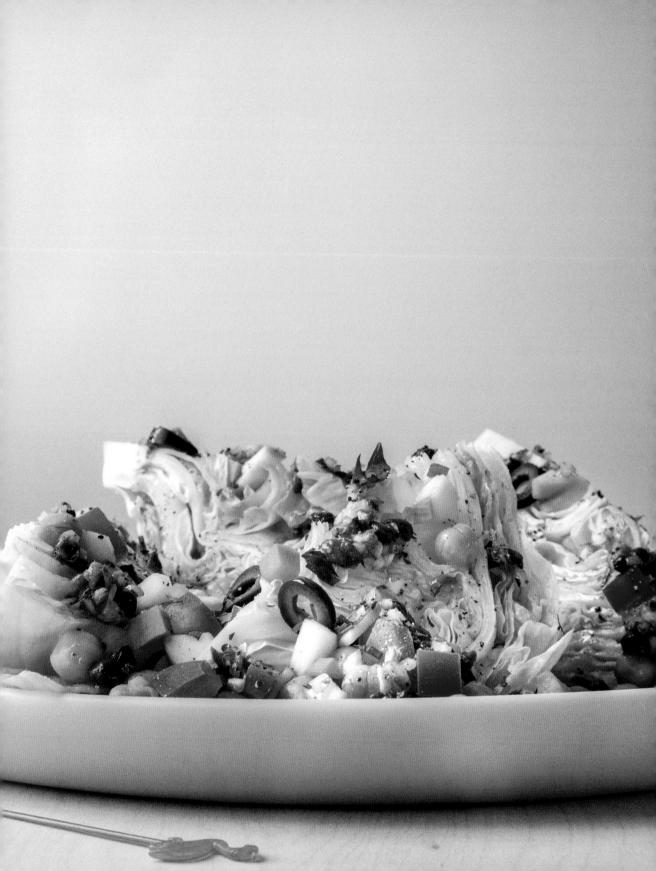

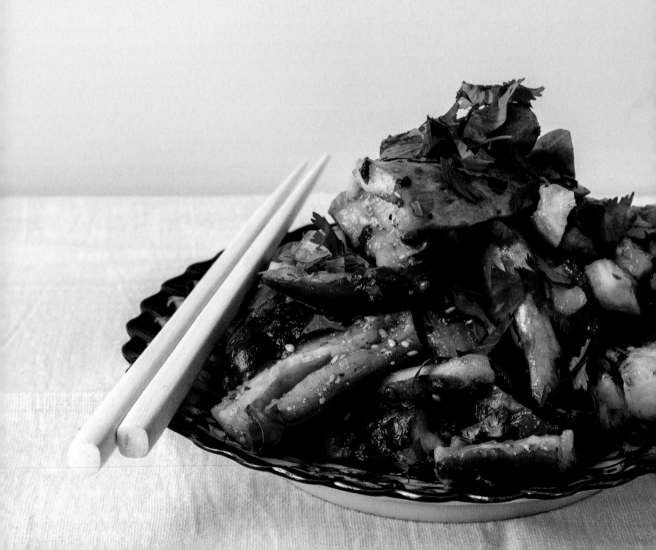

CHILI CRISP CUCUMBERS

love this salad in the summer, and the effect of mashing the cucumbers is so satisfying. The combination of the sweet juicy cucumbers and the grassy cilantro with a spicy crunch makes it a party in your mouth. If you can't source chili crisp, a hit of black pepper and cayenne will do just fine.

SERVES 2 TO 4

INGREDIENTS

6 to 8 Persian cucumbers

For the dressing

2 tablespoons tamari

2 tablespoons rice vinegar

½ teaspoon toasted sesame oil

1 teaspoon maple syrup

1 clove garlic, grated

¼ teaspoon white or black pepper

1 tablespoon sesame seeds

Garnish

1 tablespoon chili crisp, or ½ teaspoon red chili flakes

¼ cup (22 g) fresh cilantro, chopped

METHOD

Cut the cucumbers into thirds. Using the bottom of a mason jar or a masher, forcefully smash the cucumbers and transfer them to a large bowl. In a second separate bowl, whisk all the dressing ingredients together. Pour the dressing over the cucumbers and toss. Garnish with the chili crisp and cilantro.

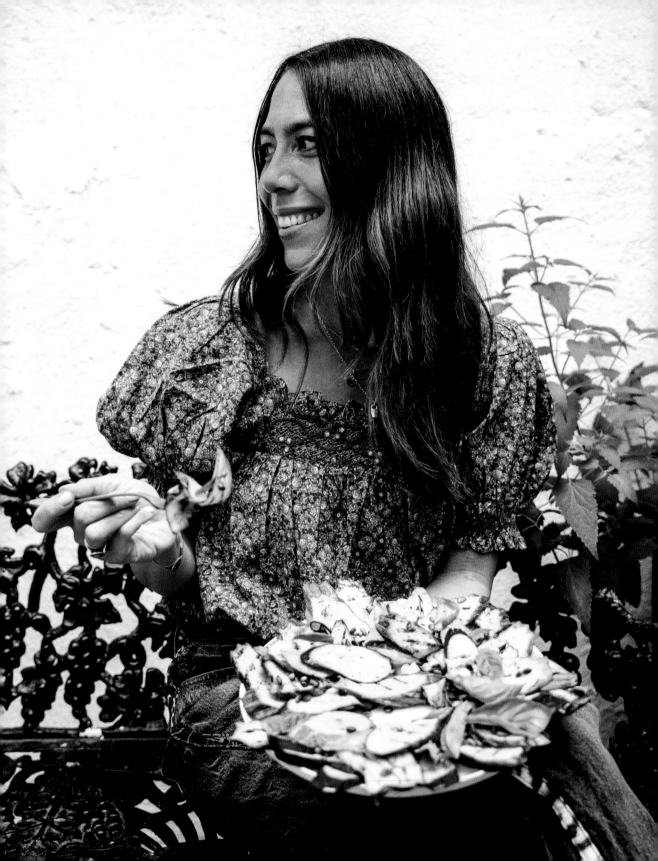

NEUTRAL VEGETABLES

HYDRATED SEAWEED

Seaweed is packed with nutrients and has been used for years in Asia as a healing ingredient, particularly after giving birth or during physical recovery. The packages of dehydrated seaweeds in the health food store or Asian market can look intimidating, but seaweeds really are the simplest thing to make, and they are wonderful as additions to salads or soups or as dishes in their own right.

SERVES 1 TO 2 PEOPLE

INGREDIENTS

½ cup dried arame or dried wakame seaweed

1 teaspoon toasted sesame oil

1 tablespoon tamari

METHOD

In a bowl, combine the seaweed and 1 cup (240 ml) water. Let soak for 20 to 30 minutes. Strain the water and, using kitchen scissors, cut the seaweed into bite-size pieces. Add the oil and tamari and massage well. The seaweed will keep in the fridge in an airtight container for up to 3 days.

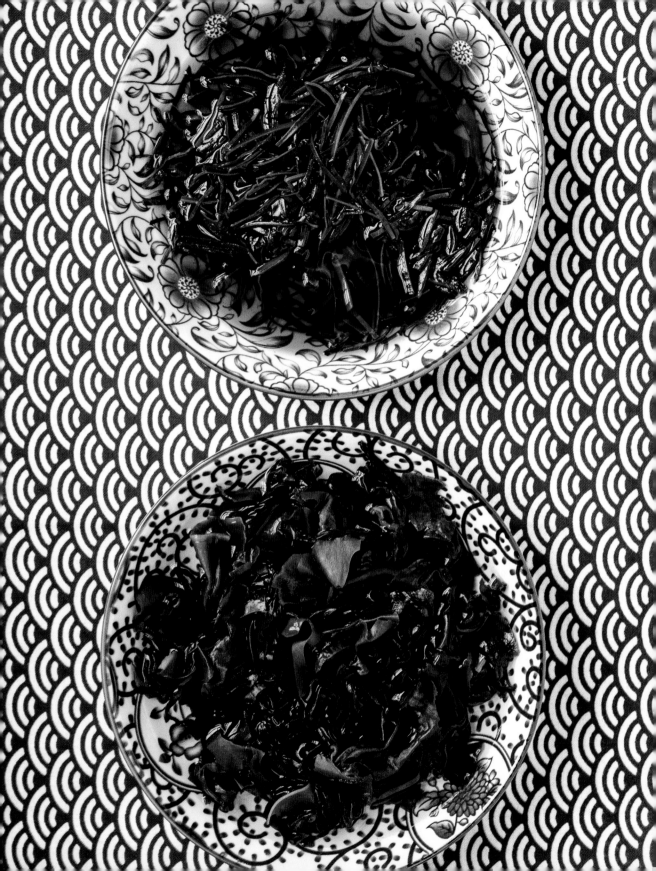

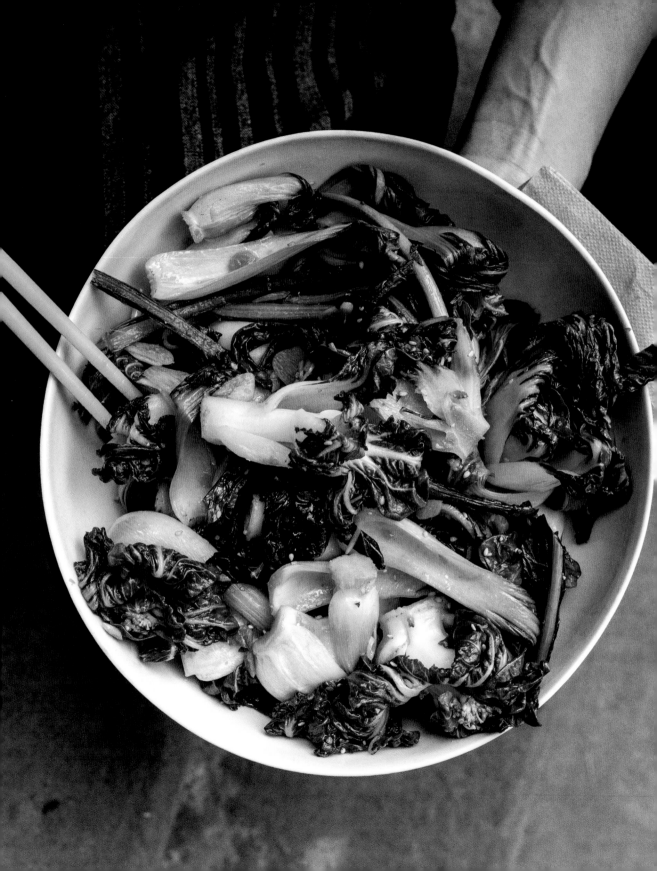

ASIAN STREET CART–STYLE GREENS

This recipe reminds me of night markets in Phuket. There are so many bustling carts to choose from—red bean-infused rice cakes, velvety mango and sticky rice, bubbling noodle soups, and exotic prickly fruits. But the ones that I try to re-create at home again and again are the humble sautéed greens that usually come as a side but are glorious on their own. Crunchy and flecked with ginger, they are truly great as a side with any meal, or serve yourself some with a heap of rice for a simple grounding meal.

SERVES 2 TO 4

INGREDIENTS

2 tablespoons avocado oil

6 cloves garlic, roughly chopped

1 teaspoon grated ginger

1 head (6½ ounces/185 g) baby bok choy, leaves separated

2 cups (70 g) destemmed and roughly chopped dandelion greens

2 cups (4 ounces/115 g) destemmed and roughly chopped lacinato kale

1 bunch (2 ounces/55 g) broccolini, trimmed and sliced lengthwise

2 tablespoons tamari

1 teaspoon rice vinegar

1 teaspoon toasted sesame oil

Garnish

1 teaspoon sesame seeds

Sea salt

Freshly ground black pepper

1 lime, quartered

METHOD

Heat a large shallow pan. Add the oil, garlic, and ginger and sauté on medium-low heat for 1 minute. Add the bok choy, dandelion greens, kale, broccolini, and tamari and sauté on high for 1 minute. Add ¼ cup (60 ml) water and continue to cook on high for 2 minutes. Cover the pan and reduce the heat to low, cooking for 1 to 2 minutes more. Remove the lid and increase the heat to cook down any remaining liquid. You want your greens bright and crunchy but cooked. Add the vinegar and sesame oil and toss. Transfer the greens to a serving plate and garnish with the sesame seeds, salt and pepper to taste, and a lime wedge.

BROILED MISO EGGPLANT

This is probably the most decadent of my recipes, simply because it's so incredibly luscious. It took me a few tries to replicate, but I think I've gotten pretty close. Although the recipe involves a few steps, the reward is a perfectly molten-hot, crisp, umami flavor bomb that makes the perfect side dish or main event with a bowl of rice.

SERVES 2 TO 4

INGREDIENTS

1 large eggplant (25¾ ounces/730 g), sliced into spears 3 to 5 inches (7.5 to 12 cm) long, or 2 Japanese eggplants, sliced lengthwise

1 to 2 tablespoons avocado oil

Sea salt

For the glaze

2 heaping tablespoons white miso paste

2 tablespoons maple syrup

2 tablespoons rice vinegar

2 tablespoons tamari

3-inch (7.5 cm) knob ginger, or 1 teaspoon grated ginger

1 clove garlic

½ small onion (4¾ ounces/135 g), grated

Garnish

2 tablespoons chopped cilantro

2 scallions, chopped

1 tablespoon sesame seeds or gomasio

METHOD

To make the eggplant: Preheat the oven to broil. Generously salt the eggplant and let sit for 15 to 20 minutes, until it begins to sweat. Pat dry with a dish towel. Using a sharp paring knife, score each side of each spear. If using smaller eggplants or Japanese eggplant, score each flesh side a few times.

Heat a skillet to medium high and add the oil. Sear each spear or side of the eggplant for 1 minute on each side, for about 3 to 4 minutes total, or until tender and slightly browned. Lower the heat, if needed: You want the eggplant to have a gold-en-brown crust; you don't want it to burn. Add more oil and a little water, if needed. Once the eggplant is browned, remove it from the heat and transfer it to a plate to cool.

To make the glaze: In a medium bowl, combine the miso, syrup, vinegar, and tamari. Using a Microplane, grate the ginger, garlic, and onion into the bowl. Whisk vigorously until a glaze forms. Transfer the eggplant to a baking dish and pour the glaze over the spears. Use a brush to distribute the glaze evenly.

Place the dish of glazed eggplant under the broiler for 3 to 5 minutes (or longer, depending on how strong your oven is). The eggplant should be bubbly and browned but not burned. Watch it carefully. Let cool slightly and garnish with the cilantro, scallions, and sesame seeds. Serve hot.

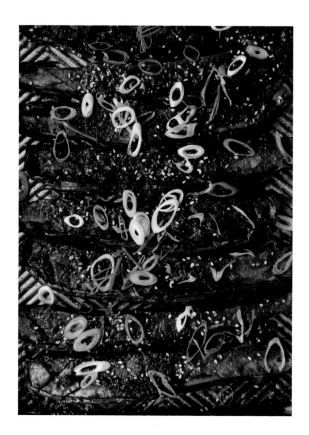

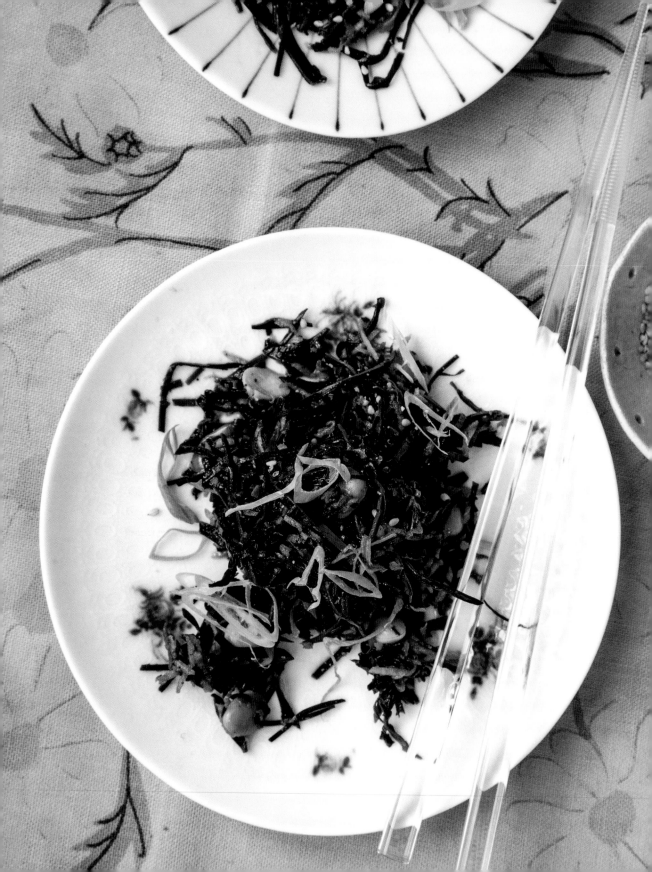

ARAME SEAWEED SALAD

This nutrient-dense salad is so comforting and cleansing at the same time. It reminds me of the dark seaweed salad that they serve at Korean restaurants in tiny banchan bowls that you always want more of. The addition of edamame beans makes it slightly heartier and a good source of plant-based protein.

SERVES 2 TO 4

INGREDIENTS

1 cup hydrated arame seaweed (5 ounces/150 g)

1 cup frozen edamame beans, defrosted

½ cup peeled and shaved carrots

½ cup thinly sliced Persian cucumbers

Dressing

4 tablespoons tamari sauce

2 tablespoons rice vinegar

1 tablespoon toasted sesame oil

½ teaspoon maple syrup

1 teaspoon toasted sesame seeds

2 scallions, thinly sliced

METHOD

Combine all salad ingredients in a medium-sized bowl. In a separate smaller bowl, whisk together the dressing ingredients. Pour the dressing over the salad and toss. Serve cold.

SPICY ROASTED BROCCOLI

This is my favorite way to eat broccoli—slightly charred, with a bite and a little kick of heat. It also takes almost no time. I could easily have this dish every single day and be perfectly happy.

SERVES 2 TO 4

INGREDIENTS

4 small bunches (3¼ pounds/1.5 kg) broccoli, stems intact

½ teaspoon garlic powder

½ teaspoon chili flakes

Dash of sea salt

Dash of freshly cracked black pepper

2 to 3 tablespoons avocado oil

For serving (optional)

Ranch Dressing (page 222) or Tahini Green Goddess Dressing (page 221)

METHOD

Preheat the oven to 400°F (205°C). Trim the ends of the broccoli stems and peel off the rough outer layer. Retaining about 3-inch (7.5-cm) stems, slice each head of broccoli lengthwise, about ¼ inch (6 mm) thick, and transfer to a large bowl. In a separate small bowl, combine the garlic powder, chili flakes, salt, and pepper. Sprinkle the spice mixture and the oil over the broccoli and massage well with your hands. On a parchment-lined baking sheet, roast the broccoli for 25 minutes, or until browned and tender. Serve with ranch or tahini green goddess dressing as a dip, if you wish.

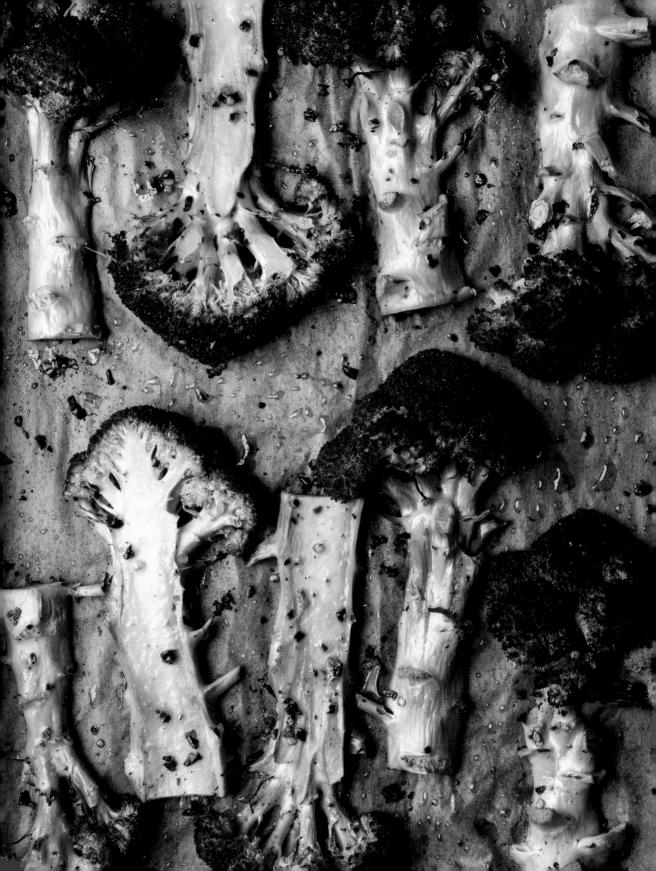

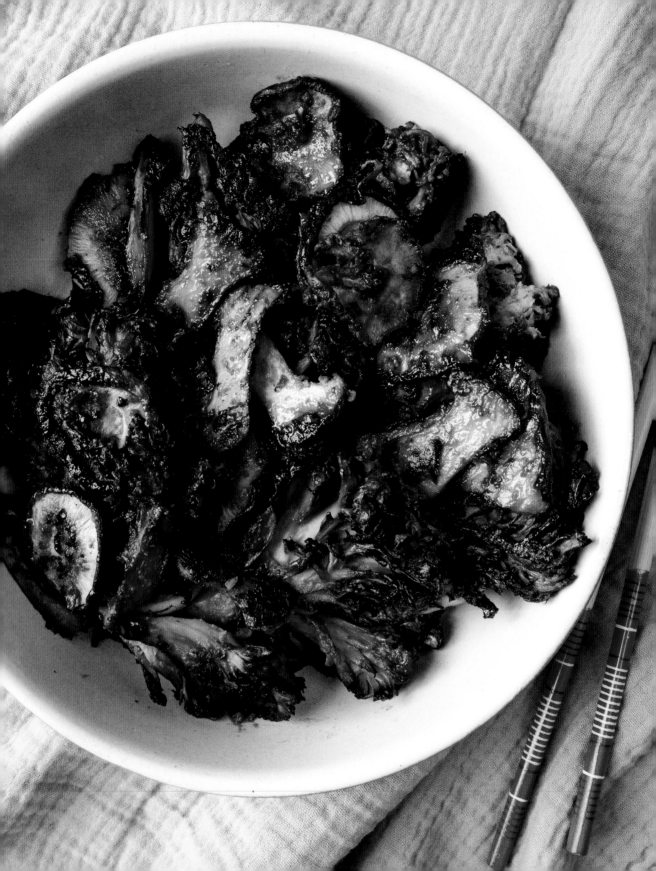

KOREAN BBQ MUSHROOMS

I grew up on Korean BBQ. To this day, the aroma of salty-sweet, crispy charred bits of bulgogi and kalbi still makes my mouth water. This recipe is the perfect dupe, especially if you can find maitake mushrooms, which crisp up perfectly and are honestly pretty, well, meaty. Dare I say it's my favorite recipe in the book?

SERVES 2 TO 4

INGREDIENTS

2 cups (100 g) shiitake mushrooms

2 cups (170 g) trumpet mushrooms

2 cups (100 g) maitake mushrooms

¼ cup (60 ml) plus 2 tablespoons Beet Gochujang (page 235) or store-bought gochujang

1 tablespoon toasted sesame oil

1 tablespoon avocado oil

Garnish

Sesame seeds or gomasio

For serving (optional)

Green or red leaf lettuce leaves

2 tablespoons miso paste

Kimchi

METHOD

Preheat the oven to 400°F (205°C). Massage the shiitake, trumpet, and maitake mushrooms with the gochujang. Transfer to a parchment-lined baking sheet and drizzle the oil on top. Roast for 20 minutes, or until browned. Sprinkle with the sesame seeds and serve with lettuce, miso paste, and kimchi, if using.

Note: I love shiitake, trumpet, maitake, and enoki mushrooms for this recipe, but feel free to sub 6 to 7 cups (370g–420g) of your favorite assortment of mushrooms.

ROASTED ARTICHOKES WITH CAPER AIOLI

This is probably one of the most time-consuming recipes in the book, but it's well worth the work. Artichokes were in regular rotation at my home. My dad would typically have one steamed whole, with a simple lemon vinaigrette to dip it in. This is a slightly more sinful version, crisped up with a creamy dipping sauce, but equally rewarding with every bite.

SERVES 4 TO 6

INGREDIENTS

4 large artichokes (3 pounds/1.36 kg)

12 cups (2.8 L) ice water

1 lemon

2 teaspoons salt

4 cloves garlic, minced

1 teaspoon sea salt

Freshly cracked black pepper

2 tablespoons avocado oil

1 cup (235 ml) Caper Aioli (recipe follows)

CAPER AIOLI

MAKES 1 CUP (235 ML)

INGREDIENTS

1 cup (240 ml) Aquafaba Mayo (page 223) or 1 (15-ounce/450-ml) jar vegan mayo

1 teaspoon Dijon mustard

1 cup (20 g) chopped chives

1 teaspoon lemon zest

Juice of 1 lemon

3 cloves garlic, grated

¼ cup (30 g) capers

Sea salt

Freshly cracked black pepper

METHOD

Preheat the oven to 450°F (230°C). Using a sharp knife, trim about ½ inch (12 mm) off the artichoke stems. With kitchen scissors, snip the sharp ends of the leaves. Fill a large bowl with the ice water. Halve the lemon and squeeze the juice into the bowl and leave the lemon halves in the water. Add the artichokes to the bowl and let sit for 15 minutes.

Meanwhile in a large pot, add the salt to 10 cups (2.4 L) water and bring to a boil. Carefully transfer the

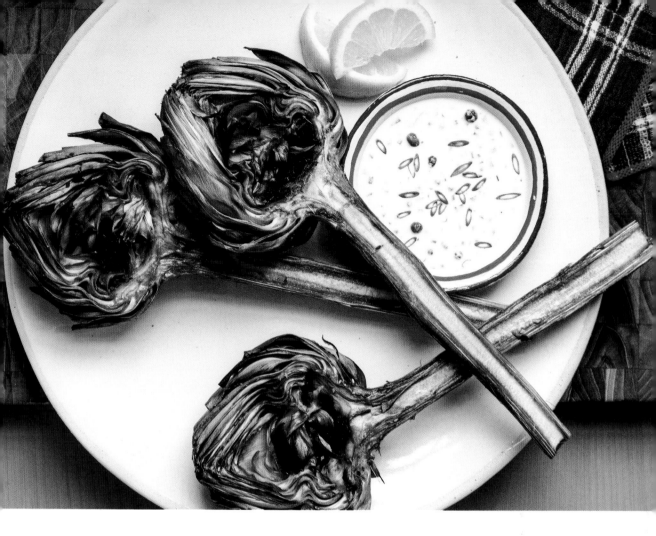

artichoke halves to the boiling water. (You may need to do this in batches, transferring 4 halves at a time.) Boil the artichokes for 8 to 10 minutes, until tender. With tongs, transfer the artichokes from the pot to a large baking sheet to cook, face up. Sprinkle the garlic evenly into the cavities of the artichokes and season with the sea salt and pepper to taste. Drizzle the oil evenly on the artichokes and roast for 15 to 20 minutes, until browned and crisp.

While the artichokes are roasting, make the caper aioli: In a medium bowl, combine the mayo, mustard, chives, lemon zest, lemon juice, garlic, and capers until well blended. Season with salt and pepper to taste. Serve in a small bowl or ramekin for dipping.

BUFFALO CAULIFLOWER

Hot, sticky, and sweet, this dish was born out of Superbowl Sunday, but it can certainly be enjoyed away from the couch. Serve it, ideally, with ranch dressing as a dipping sauce, because it's impossible to imagine Buffalo anything without ranch.

SERVES 2

INGREDIENTS

1 head cauliflower, or 4 cups florets (18 ounces/505 g)

⅓ cup (75 ml) Bonberi Hot Sauce (page 225) or your favorite red hot sauce

½ teaspoon ground cumin

1 teaspoon garlic powder

1 teaspoon onion powder

½ teaspoon smoked paprika

2 to 3 tablespoons avocado oil

For serving

Ranch Dressing (page 222)

METHOD

Preheat the oven to 425°F (220°C). Break the cauliflower into bite-size florets and place them in a baking pan. In a small bowl, whisk the hot sauce, cumin, garlic powder, onion powder, paprika, and oil. Pour the mixture over the cauliflower and, using a spatula, coat well. (If using your hands, wear gloves.) Roast for 30 minutes, until browned and crisp. Let cool and serve with the ranch dressing.

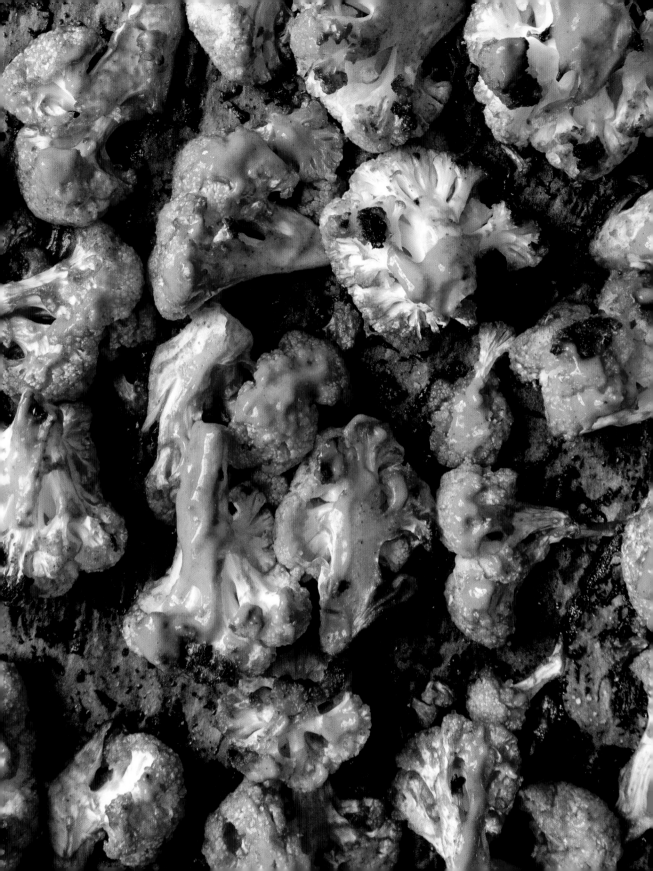

SZECHUAN EGGPLANT AND BEANS

This dish is a tribute to the Chinese American restaurants I grew up with in New Jersey. Using corn starch to crisp up the eggplant makes it taste decadent, and whenever I'm craving that throwback take-out meal, this is what I make, with some short-grain rice.

SERVES 2

INGREDIENTS

1 medium eggplant (4 cups/345 g), chopped into ½-inch (12-mm) cubes

2 tablespoons avocado oil

1 teaspoon sea salt

2 cloves garlic, minced

2 tablespoons tamari

1 tablespoon rice vinegar

½ teaspoon coconut sugar

1 tablespoon toasted sesame oil

½ teaspoon white or black pepper

½ teaspoon chili flakes or thinly sliced red chili pepper

2 cups (250 g) green beans, trimmed

1 teaspoon toasted sesame seeds or gomasio

Garnish

2 scallions, thinly sliced

Optional

2 teaspoons cornstarch

METHOD

On a dish towel, lay the eggplant cubes flat and generously salt them. Let sit to sweat for 15 to 20 minutes.

In a large frying pan or wok, heat the avocado oil. Add the garlic and sauté on medium heat for 1 to 2 minutes, until fragrant. Pat the eggplant dry with a towel and, in a large bowl, sprinkle the cornstarch, if using, over the cubes until they are fully coated. Add the eggplant to the pan and sauté for 5 to 6 minutes. You might need to add a little water to prevent sticking.

Once the eggplant is cooked, leave in the pan and slide off heat. In a bowl, whisk together the tamari, vinegar, sugar, sesame oil, white pepper, chili flakes, and sesame seeds.

Return to the cooked eggplant, add the beans to the pan, and pour in the tamari mixture. Bring the pan to a high heat, adding more water if needed to prevent sticking, and continue to stir but allow the eggplant and beans to brown. Garnish with sliced scallions.

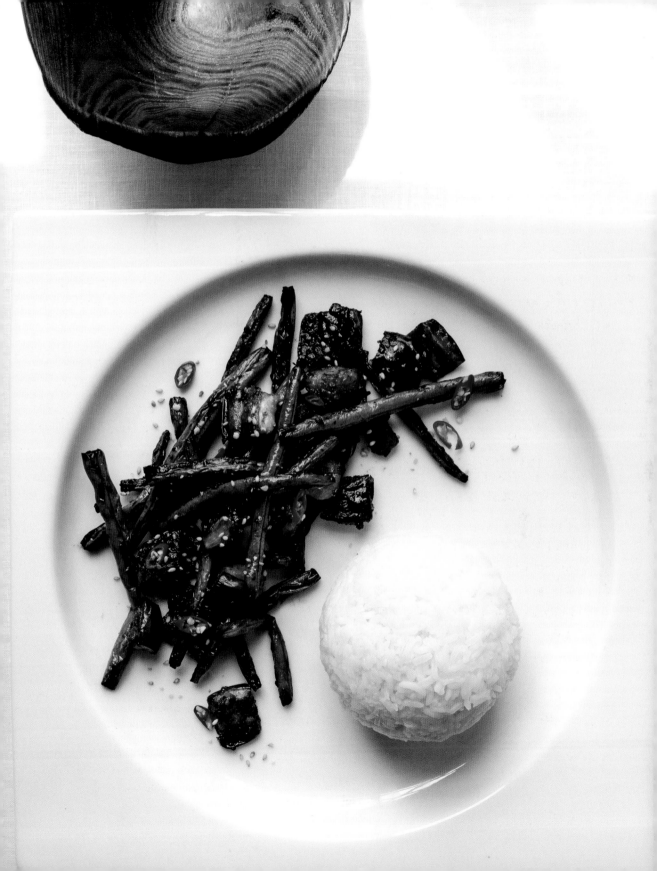

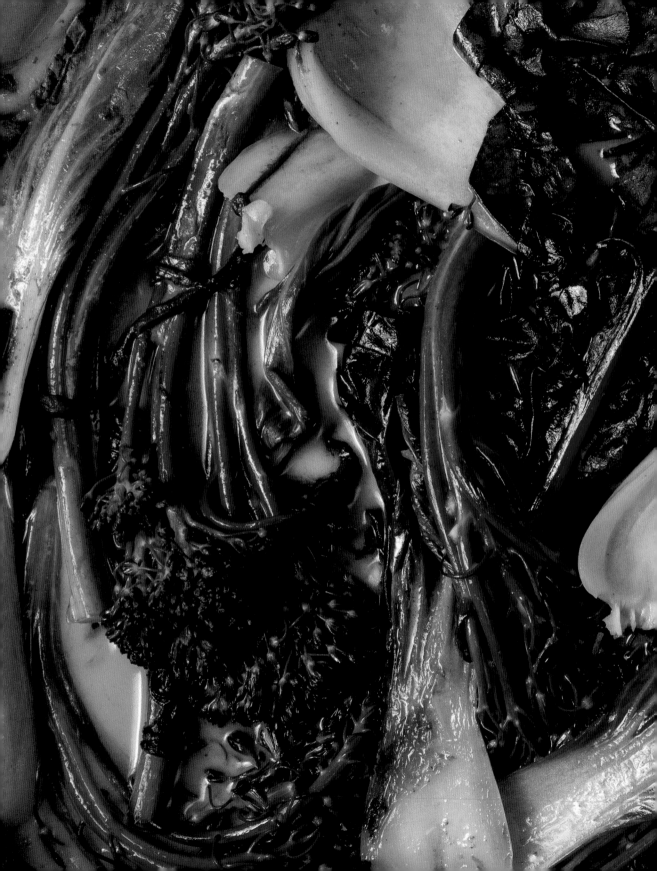

BROTHY TURMERIC GREENS

I love this dish because you can make it in less than 15 minutes and it's incredibly grounding and satisfying yet also cleansing. You can get creative, using whatever veggies you have in the fridge, and serve it with rice or keep it grain-free.

SERVES 1 TO 2

INGREDIENTS

1 to 2 tablespoons coconut oil or avocado oil

1 clove garlic, minced

1 teaspoon grated ginger

½ teaspoon ground turmeric

1 bunch broccolini, sliced lengthwise

2 bunches baby bok choy, pulled apart

1 can (13½-ounce/398-g) unsweetened coconut milk

1 teaspoon coconut sugar

Sea salt

Freshly cracked black pepper

For serving (optional)

Brown or purple rice

METHOD

In a large shallow pan, heat the oil. Add the garlic and ginger, and a little water to prevent sticking. Add the turmeric and sauté on medium-high heat. Season with salt and pepper to taste. Add the broccolini and continue sautéing. Once the broccolini is bright green, add the bok choy and a little more water (don't add more than a total of ½ cup/ 120 ml water; you don't want the dish too brothy) and steam, covered, for only a couple of minutes. Remove the lid and add the coconut milk and sugar and combine. Remove the pan from the heat. Spoon the greens into a shallow bowl and serve with rice, if using.

SALT-AND-PEPPER MUSHROOMS

This is an unbelievably simple recipe that I return to time and again. What makes this dish, in my opinion, is the combination of the fiery black pepper and the mixed varieties of mushrooms. Note: If you cannot find the specific mushroom varietals below, feel free to use whatever you can find!

SERVES 2 TO 4

INGREDIENTS

4 king trumpet mushrooms (10¾ ounces/305 g), stems removed and sliced diagonally, about ⅛ inch (3 mm) thick (see Note)

2 cups (175 g) shiitake mushroom caps, sliced about ⅛ inch (3 mm) thick

2 cups (150 g) shimeji mushrooms, stems removed and sliced about ⅛ inch (3 mm) thick

2 tablespoons avocado oil

2 cloves garlic, minced

½ teaspoon sea salt

Freshly cracked black pepper

Juice of ½ lemon

Optional

1 tablespoon grass-fed butter, ghee, or vegan butter

Garnish

1 bunch chives, finely chopped

1 lemon wedge

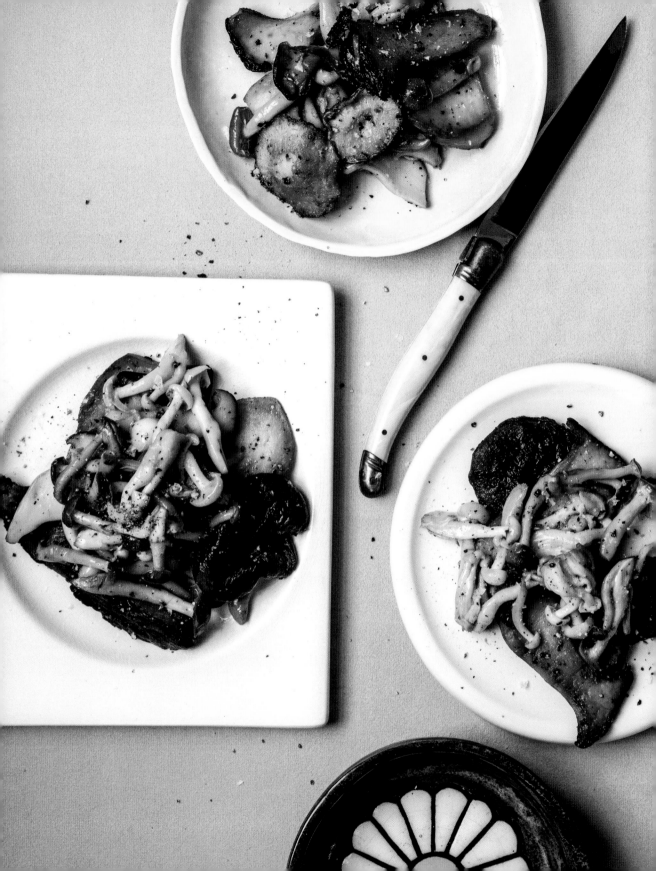

METHOD

In a large bowl, combine the king trumpet, shii-take, and shimeji mushrooms. In a large shallow saucepan, heat the oil on medium high. Add the garlic and sauté for about 3 minutes, until fragrant but not browned. Add the mushrooms in batches and begin to sauté on high. Add ½ teaspoon of salt and a generous amount of pepper. Add ¼ cup (60 ml) water to help cook down the mushrooms, if needed.

Do not cover the pan. Let the mushrooms sit for a few minutes to help brown the ends. Stir occasionally, scraping the pan to prevent burning. If the mushrooms begin to brown too quickly, add more water or lower the heat. Continue to sauté, 7 to 8 minutes, stirring only occasionally, scraping the bottom, and watching the heat. Once the mushrooms have cooked down, add the butter, if using, and season with more salt and pepper, as needed. Turn off the heat, squeeze in lemon juice, and toss. Transfer to a serving bowl and top with the chives and lemon wedge. Serve immediately.

Note: If you can't source king trumpet, shiitake, and shimeji mushrooms, any assortment will do. I find it nice to combine at least three varieties of mushrooms, with different textures and meatiness. Save and freeze the mushroom stems for Vegan Dashi Broth (page 157).

BEET TARTARE

This dish is meant for presentation and entertaining. You could definitely make it just for yourself, but there is a refinement to it and a fun way of serving it that will certainly please guests. It's inspired by the steak tartare from famed brasserie Bofinger, in Paris's 4th arrondissement, which is a dish my friends would often order, and it was my goal to make a plant-based version. Instead of a classic raw egg yolk, I've created a creamy, herby dressing that lends an almost "yolk-y" creaminess that could certainly double as a yummy salad dressing or dip.

SERVES 2 TO 4

INGREDIENTS

For the beets

2 large red beets (9½ ounces/270 g), quartered

4 small golden beets
(7½ ounces/210 g), halved

1 large candy cane beet
(9½ ounces/270 g), quartered

½ cup (100 g) celery, finely chopped

¼ cup (30 g) capers

For the dressing

¼ cup (60 ml) Aquafaba Mayo
(page 223)

2 tablespoons olive oil

1 tablespoon fresh lemon juice

2 tablespoons apple cider vinegar

2 tablespoons tamari

1 shallot, minced (1½ ounces/45 g)

2 tablespoons chopped fresh dill

2 tablespoons chopped fresh parsley

Sea salt

Freshly cracked black pepper

For serving

Kettle-cooked potato chips

Two Belgian endives, separated into leaves

2 tablespoons of Aquafaba Mayo (page 223) or store-bought vegan mayo

METHOD

Make the beets: Fill a large pot fitted with a steamer basket with 1 to 2 inches (2½ to 5 cm) water and bring to a boil. Place the red, golden, and candy cane beets in the basket, cover the pot, and let steam for about 20 minutes, until the beets are tender. Remove the beets from the steamer and let cool for 10 minutes, then peel them.

One color at a time, chop the beets into small cubes and place them in separate bowls.

Make the dressing: In a bowl, stir the mayo, oil, lemon juice, vinegar, tamari, shallot, dill, and parsley until well combined.

Pour one-third of the dressing into each bowl of beets and combine well. Season with salt and pepper, if needed. Transfer each beet mixture to a large ramekin or serving bowl and gently combine. Then pack the ramekin tightly and place a flat plate on top of it. Flip the plate over while keeping the ramekin tight against the plate's surface. Carefully lift the ramekin to release. Serve with the potato chips and/or endive.

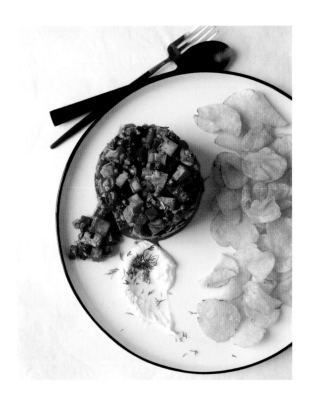

VEGETABLE BANCHAN

The best part about eating out at Korean restaurants is banchan, the small delicious plates they set in front of you are a meal in their own right! When I was little, I would delight in crunching my way through salty zucchini, tender bean sprouts, and melt-in-your mouth radish, not realizing how naturally plant-based Korean meals are. Below are my top three that may seem intimidating at first but truly simple to make.

BEAN SPROUT BANCHAN

SERVES 2 TO 4

INGREDIENTS

1 teaspoon salt

4 heaping cups (395 g) mung bean sprouts

2 teaspoons toasted sesame oil

1 tablespoon rice vinegar

2 cloves garlic, grated

2 tablespoons toasted sesame seeds or gomasio

Sea salt

Freshly cracked black pepper

METHOD

In a medium saucepan, add the salt to 6 cups (1.5 L) water and bring to a boil. Add the bean sprouts and boil for 5 minutes. Drain and let cool. Transfer the sprouts to a medium bowl. Add the oil, vinegar, garlic, and sesame seeds. Massage well. Season with more salt and pepper, if needed. Serve with rice or as a side dish.

ZUCCHINI BANCHAN

SERVES 2 TO 4

INGREDIENTS

6 small zucchini, thinly sliced or shaved into coins (7 cups/1 kg)

1 teaspoon salt

2 teaspoons toasted sesame oil

2 cloves garlic, grated

1 teaspoon maple syrup

Dash of cayenne pepper

1 teaspoon sesame seeds

Optional

2 tablespoons dulse flakes

METHOD

On a dish towel, lay the zucchini coins flat. Sprinkle the salt evenly over them and let sit for 30 minutes or up to an hour. Bring the ends of the towel together to form a pouch and, over the sink, wring out the towel with the zucchini inside super tightly to release the excess liquid. Make sure you squeeze well to release as much liquid as possible. Transfer the drained zucchini to a medium bowl.

In small bowl, whisk together the oil, garlic, syrup, cayenne, sesame seeds, and dulse flakes (if using). Pour over the drained zucchini and massage well. Serve with rice or as a side dish.

DAIKON RADISH BANCHAN

SERVES 2 TO 4

INGREDIENTS

1 daikon radish (14 ounces/391g) peeled and cubed into ½-inch cubes (2½ cups)

1 teaspoon salt

1 teaspoon toasted sesame oil

1 tablespoon rice vinegar

1 garlic clove, grated

2 scallions, thinly sliced (1½ ounces/40g)

1 teaspoon sesame seeds

Sea salt and pepper

METHOD

Peel and cut the daikon radish into 1-inch cubes and set aside. In a medium saucepan, add the salt to 6 cups (1.5 L) water and bring to a boil. Add the daikon and boil for 5 minutes. Drain and let cool. Transfer the daikon to a medium bowl. Add the oil, vinegar, garlic, scallions, and sesame seeds and massage well. Season with more salt and pepper if needed. Serve with rice or as a side dish.

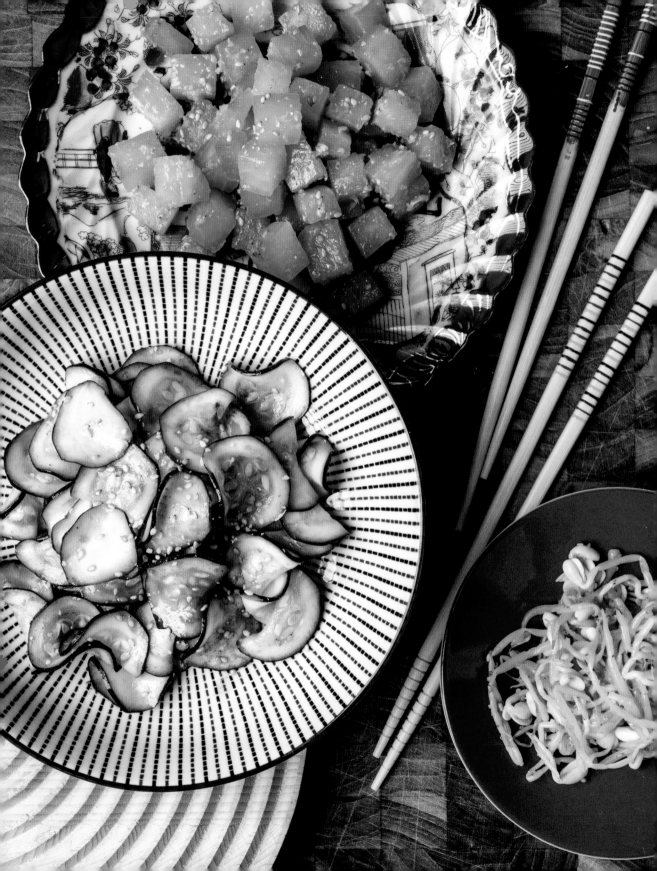

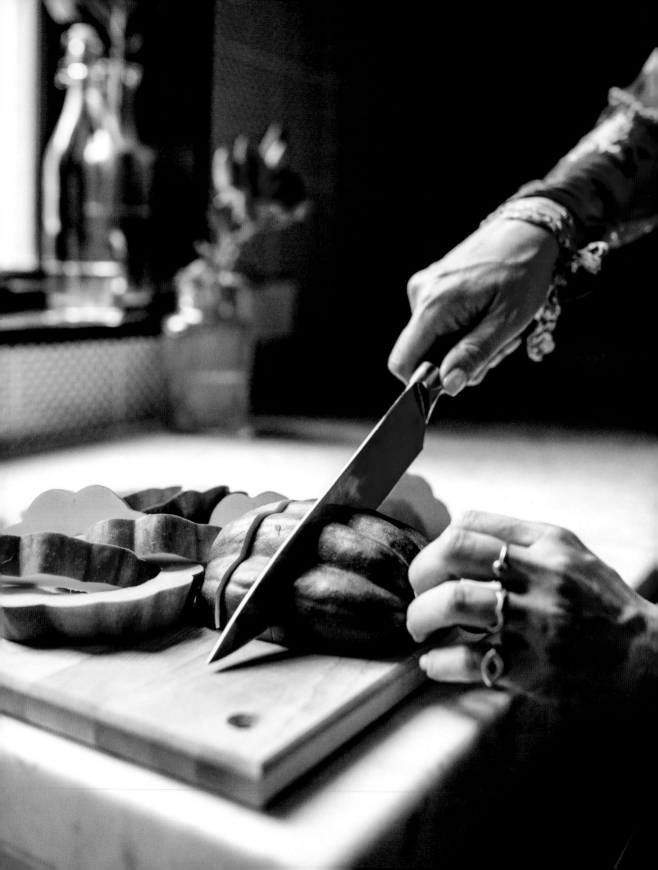

STARCHY VEGETABLES AND LEGUMES

ICE BATH POTATO FRIES

t's funny how a simple trick can really make a recipe. Enter the ice bath potatoes. I can't take full credit for the tip to shock your potatoes in a bath of ice-cold water to remove excess starch, but I can take credit for eating a boatload of perfectly crisp baked potatoes since learning said tip. My version uses russet potatoes with a little savory spice, but you can sub any white potato you want. (My kids have these seasoned only with sea salt almost every day.) The recipe doesn't work as well with sweet potatoes. So delight in the original!

SERVES 2 TO 4

INGREDIENTS

4 russet potatoes (3 pounds/1.4 kg), scrubbed

2 cups ice

Juice of ½ lemon

¼ cup (60 ml) avocado oil

1 teaspoon garlic powder

1 teaspoon paprika

1 teaspoon onion powder

1 tablespoon dried oregano

1 teaspoon sea salt

Pinch of black pepper

METHOD

Preheat the oven to 400°F (205°C).

Keeping the skin on the potatoes (if you prefer the skin off—for classic fries— that works too!), slice off the ends. Then slice the potatoes lengthwise into quarters, and slice the quarters into wedges. Make sure the wedges are all roughly the same size.

Fill a large bowl halfway with water, the ice, and lemon juice. Lemon juice prevents potatoes from browning. Add the potatoes and let sit, fully submerged in the ice water, for 20 minutes or up to an hour.

Drain the potatoes and lay them out on a dish towel to dry. Clean the bowl and return the potatoes to it. Add the oil, garlic powder, paprika, onion powder, oregano, salt, and pepper and massage well with your hands.

Arrange the potatoes on a parchment-lined baking sheet. Roast for 30 to 35 minutes, until tender and crisped at the edges. Let cool a bit and enjoy!

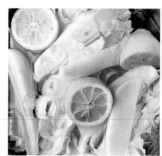

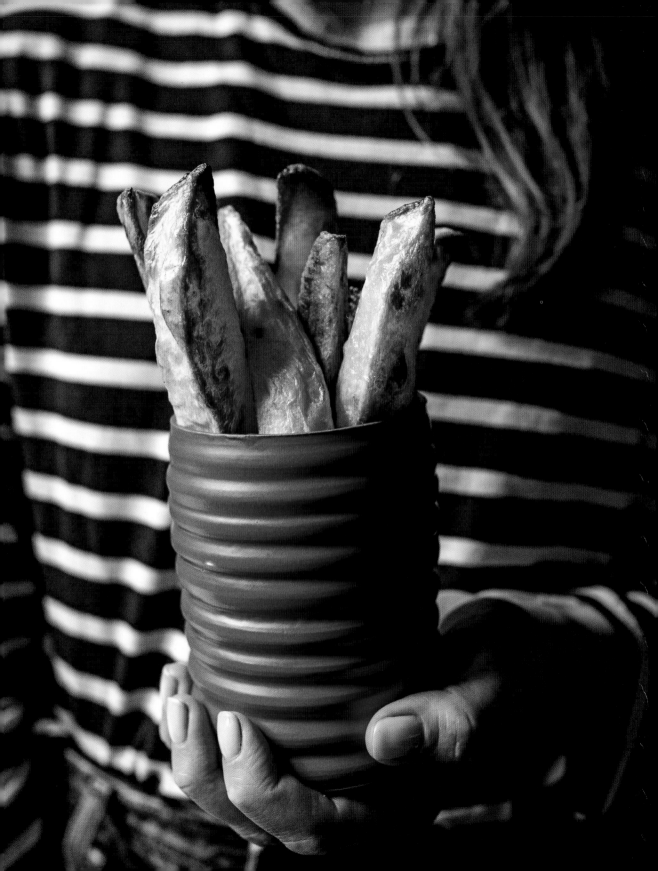

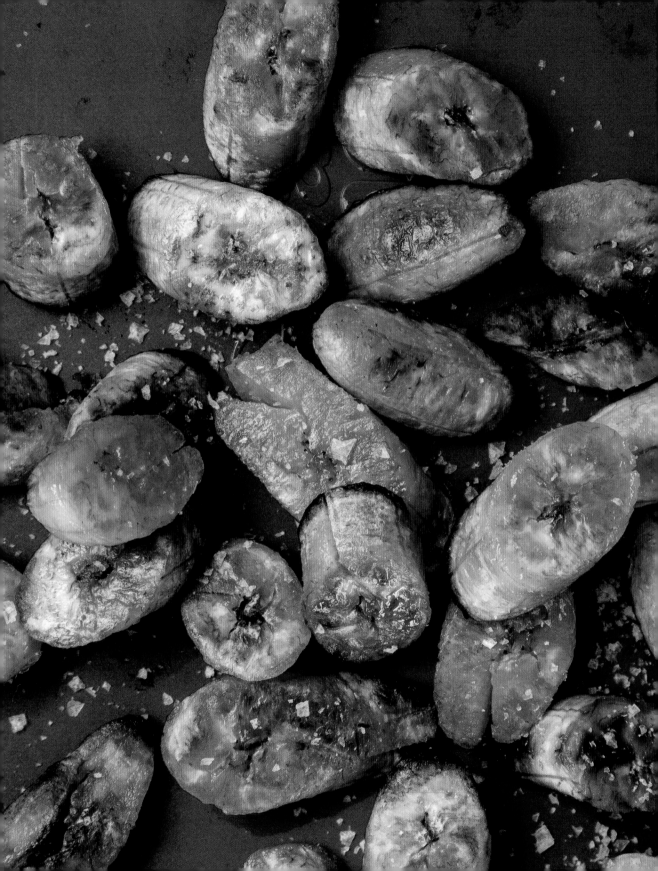

BAKED CARAMELIZED PLANTAINS

I was admittedly late to the platanos game, but oh so happy I got here. I have to credit my friend Paola for teaching me how she makes her sweet plantains. This method is how I make them as crisp and succulent as the deep-fried versions you find at restaurants.

SERVES 2

INGREDIENTS

4 plantains (2 pounds/1 kg), ripe and spotted but firm

2 tablespoons avocado oil

½ teaspoon sea salt

¼ teaspoon black pepper, or a few twists of freshly cracked black pepper

Optional

Flaky sea salt

METHOD

Preheat the oven to 375°F (190°C)—or 400°F/205°C, if your oven runs cool. Slice off both ends of the plantains. With a sharp knife, make one slit lengthwise into the peel of each plantain. With your hands, pull the peels off, keeping the plantains intact. Slice them into rounds ¾ inch (2 cm) thick.

Line a 9½ by 13-inch (24 by 33-cm) or larger baking sheet with parchment paper. Transfer the plantain rounds to the sheet. Drizzle with the oil, add the salt and pepper, and massage well with your hands until fully coated. Arrange the rounds on the sheet so that they are flat and do not overlap. Bake for 20 minutes and then, using tongs, flip the rounds. This step is essential and gives you perfectly caramelized outsides with molten soft insides like the ones you get from deep-frying. Bake for 15 minutes or so more. You want the edges to be slightly brown and caramelized. Season with flaky salt, if using. Remove the rounds from the pan and enjoy warm. (These will harden after 20 minutes or so, so I like to keep them under a dish towel or eat them right away!)

JAP CHAE

J ap Chae is a foundational dish in many Korean households and actually quite simple to make. It is basically stir-fried sweet potato glass noodles with tons of vegetables and seasoning. Traditionally served with shredded meat and egg, I actually think you don't miss a thing when it's vegetarian. The noodles are made from sweet potato starch, so it's naturally gluten and grain free. It's so simple and comforting that I make it for my family year-round.

SERVES 4

INGREDIENTS

6 ounces (170 g) dried sweet potato noodles

2 tablespoons avocado oil

1 medium yellow onion, peeled, halved, and thinly sliced

2-inch (5-cm) knob ginger, peeled and grated

1 clove garlic, minced

2 small zucchini, cut into strips ⅛ inch (3 mm) thick and 3 inches (7½ cm) long

1 head broccoli, chopped

4 medium carrots, cut into strips ⅛ inch (3 mm) thick and 3 inches (7½ cm) long

1 red bell pepper, destemmed, cored, and thinly sliced

2 cups (10½ ounces/300 g) shiitake mushroom caps, thinly sliced

6 tablespoons tamari

2 teaspoons toasted sesame oil

½ teaspoon sea salt

2 cups (60 g) packed baby spinach

Garnish

2 scallions, minced

1 teaspoon toasted sesame seeds

Optional

¼ cup store-bought vegan kimchi

For serving

2 to 4 Persian cucumbers, quartered lengthwise

1 head romaine, separated into leaves

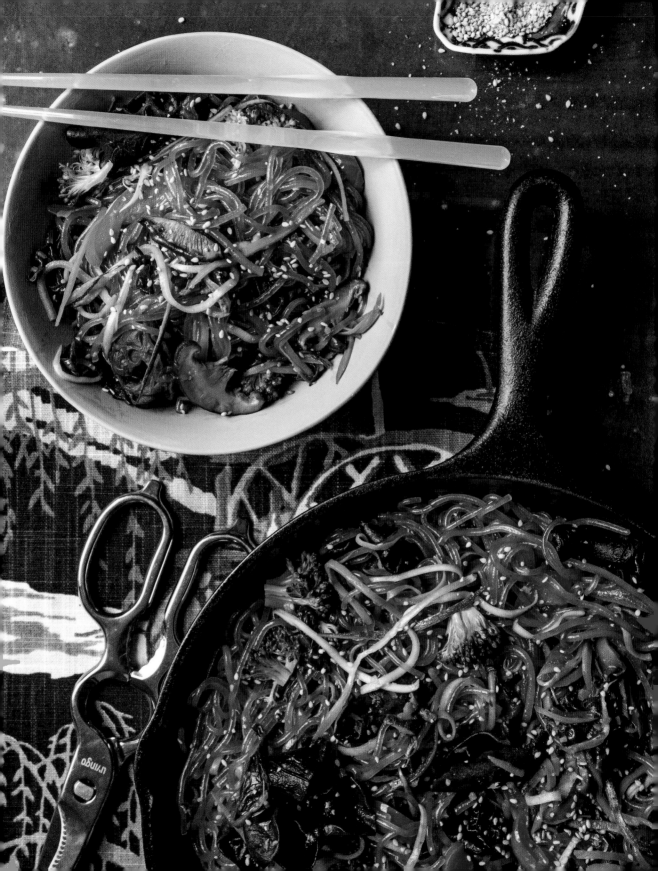

METHOD

In a saucepan, bring 6 cups (1.5 L) water to a boil, turn off the heat, and add the noodles; let sit for about 4 minutes until soft. Drain the noodles, rinse with cold water, and set aside in a bowl. If cooking noodles hours or the day before, massage with 1 teaspoon of toasted sesame oil to prevent clumping.

In a 4-quart (3.8-L) or larger pan, heat the avocado oil. Add the onion, ginger, and garlic and sauté on medium heat for 2 to 3 minutes, until the onion is soft but not browned. Add the zucchini, broccoli, carrots, pepper, mushrooms, 4 tablespoons of the tamari, 1 teaspoon of the sesame oil, and the salt. Sauté on medium high, stirring occasionally, for 5 to 7 minutes, until the vegetables are well cooked. At 5 minutes, add the spinach and gently stir in until cooked. Lower the heat to a simmer and add the noodles, gently folding them into the veggies. It helps to use tongs. Combine well on low heat for about 2 minutes. Continue to toss until the translucent noodles turn a light brown hue.

Add the remaining 2 tablespoons tamari and 1 teaspoon sesame oil and season with more salt, if needed. Using kitchen scissors, cut the noodles several times. (You can do this at the table for a more authentic effect!) Transfer the noodles to a large serving plate and garnish with the scallions, sesame seeds, and kimchi, if using. I like to serve the dish with Persian cucumbers and romaine leaves for wrapping!

You can find sweet potato starch noodles at most Asian grocers or online, but can also sub mung bean or kelp noodles here as well.

COOKING LEGUMES 101

FOR YEARS I DID NOT CONSIDER MYSELF THE soaking and stewing type of person. Too much work. Too much time. Too much preparation. Then I had kids, and the thought of purchasing aluminum cans every time I wanted them to have some plant-based protein didn't sit well. So I changed! As kids often cause us to do. Don't fret if you're still the canned type. I still use canned beans every so often, but when I do, I notice the difference in the way they taste and digest. It's worth big-batching these, so you can have them ready in your fridge to add to salads, soups, and curries whenever you please.

GENERAL TIPS FOR COOKING LEGUMES:

USE A 1:4 RATIO WHEN SOAKING. SO IF you're soaking 1 cup (200 g) dried garbanzo beans, add 4 cups (960 ml) water (the beans will expand overnight).

TYPICALLY SOAK YOUR BEANS OVERNIGHT or for 6 hours (any longer, and they will begin to sprout, which is actually a good thing for digestion, but we're talking basic beans here).

OPT FOR ORGANIC BEANS.

ADD 1 SHEET KOMBU SEAWEED AND 1 TABLE-spoon apple cider vinegar to your water. This helps make them more digestible.

USE A 1:6 RATIO WHEN COOKING. SO IF you're cooking 1 cup (250 g) dried black beans, add 6 cups (1.4 L) water.

WHEN COOKING, SEASON YOUR WATER! Many people make the mistake of cooking beans in water and just water, which makes for bland-tasting beans. I love to add a bay leaf, at least 1 teaspoon sea salt, garlic, onion, and even carrots or herbs to my water to infuse the beans with flavor.

SAVE THE COOKING LIQUID! THE LIQUID that the beans cook in is pure gold. Save it in the fridge and then add it to soups, rice, or quinoa as a flavor boost. It's a game changer.

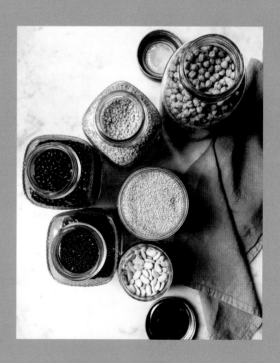

SESAME MUNG BEAN NOODLES

Sesame noodles are an unearthly delight. They're incredibly creamy and decadent but also packed with plant-based protein and perfectly combined when using glass noodles like these.

SERVES 4

INGREDIENTS

1 (6-ounce/170-g) package dried mung bean noodles or kelp noodles (see Note)

1 cup (240 ml) Peanut Sesame Dressing (recipe follows)

PEANUT SESAME DRESSING

MAKES 1 CUP (240 ML) DRESSING

INGREDIENTS

½ cup (120 ml) smooth natural peanut butter

2 teaspoons toasted sesame oil

¼ cup (60 ml) tamari

¼ cup (60 ml) rice vinegar

2 teaspoons maple syrup

1 teaspoon grated ginger

Dash of cayenne pepper

Sea salt

Garnish

4 Persian cucumbers, thinly sliced lengthwise and cut into long matchsticks

2 scallions, minced

Optional

1 teaspoon gomasio or toasted sesame seeds

For serving

1 cup (240 ml) ice cubes

METHOD

Make the noodles: In a medium saucepan, boil 4 cups (960 ml) water. Remove from heat. Add the noodles and let sit for 1 to 2 minutes until soft. Drain the noodles and rinse with cold water. Transfer the cooked noodles to a bowl, and using kitchen scissors, cut them several times. Set aside.

Make the dressing: In a medium bowl, whisk together the peanut butter, oil, tamari, vinegar, syrup, ginger, and cayenne with ¼ cup (60 ml) water until creamy. Add salt to taste. Pour the dressing over the noodles and toss.

To serve: Transfer the noodles to a serving bowl with the ice cubes at the bottom. Top with the cucumber, scallions, and gomasio, if using.

Note: For soft kelp noodles: rinse under cold water, then submerge noodles in a bowl of 3 cups (720 ml) of water, 1 tablespoon baking soda, and the juice of 1 lemon for 15 minutes. Strain and use as needed.

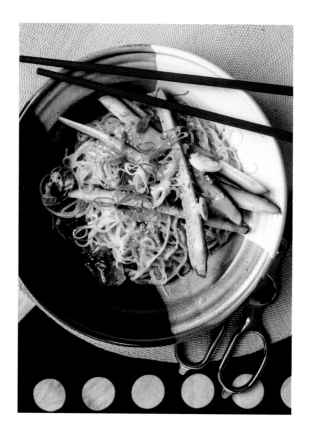

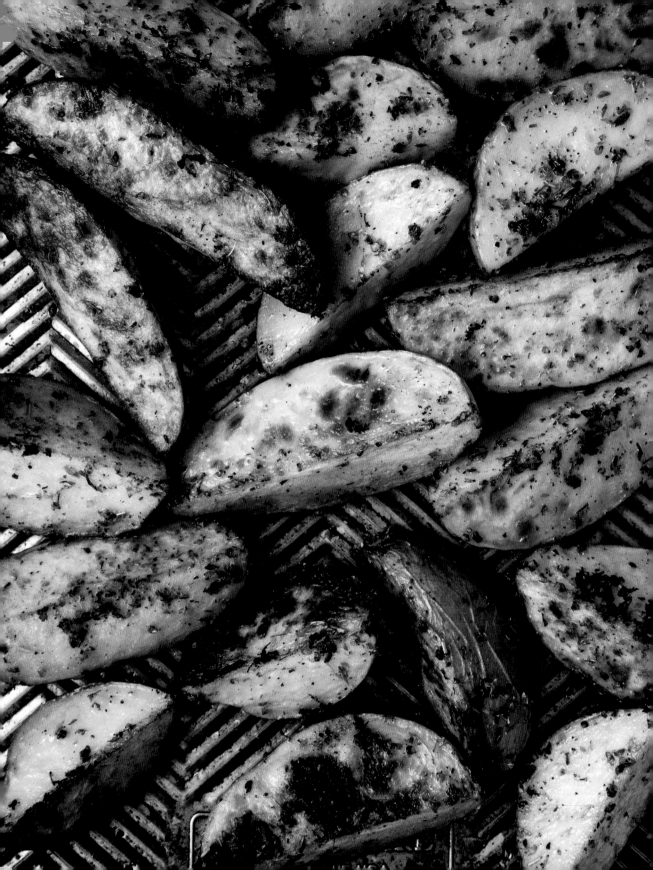

LEMONY OREGANO POTATOES

This is one of the simplest yet richest home-cooked recipes that you will come to again and again. No, the amount of lemon juice isn't a typo. You want to basically steep the potatoes in the lemon-water mixture to half bake, half stew them, resulting in the juicy yet caramelized spears that you'll have to fight over at the dinner table.

SERVES 2 TO 4

INGREDIENTS

2½ pounds (1.2 kg) Yukon gold potatoes (6 to 8 potatoes), peeled and sliced into wedges

Juice of 2 to 3 lemons, or ⅓ cup (75 ml) lemon juice

1 tablespoon dried oregano

1 teaspoon garlic powder

1 teaspoon sea salt

Freshly cracked black pepper

¼ cup (60 ml) olive oil

METHOD

Preheat the oven to 450°F (230°C). In a large bowl, combine the potatoes, lemon juice, oregano, garlic powder, salt, and pepper to taste. Massage well. Transfer to a baking dish 2 inches (5 cm) deep. (You want the dish to be large enough so that the wedges don't overlap.) Pour ⅓ cup (75 ml) water over the potatoes and drizzle the oil on top.

Roast for 20 minutes. Remove from the oven, baste with a large spoon, flip the potatoes, and roast for 20 to 25 minutes more, until golden brown with crisp edges. Let cool and serve.

SIMPLE ROASTED ACORN SQUASH

This may be one of the simpler recipes in the book, but it's one I whip out every fall and winter. With very little oil and the seasoning, the way this slightly sweet squash roasts is pure magic.

SERVES 1 TO 2 PEOPLE

INGREDIENTS

1 acorn squash (1¾ pounds/795 g), halved, seeded, and sliced into ½-inch (12-mm) thick half-moons

2 tablespoons avocado oil or coconut oil

½ teaspoon ground cinnamon

½ teaspoon coriander

½ teaspoon sea salt

METHOD

Preheat the oven to 400°F (205°C). Place the squash moons on a parchment-lined baking sheet. Sprinkle them with the oil, cinnamon, coriander, and salt and massage well with your hands. Roast for 20 minutes, or until browned. Enjoy immediately.

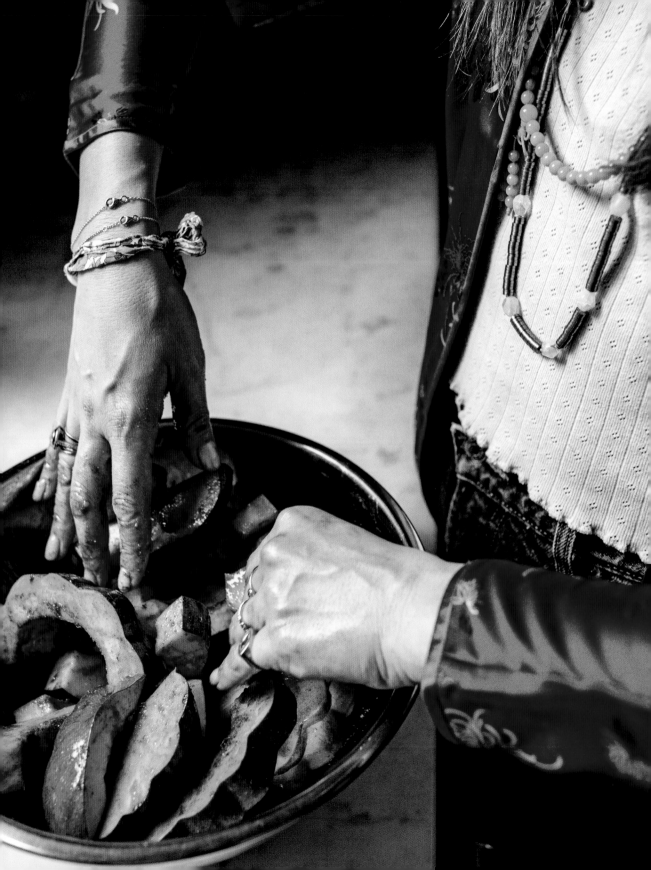

UNI'S MUNG BEAN PANCAKES

This is my mother's recipe, so I can't take any credit. I've texted her time and again to get the recipe right, and still my pancakes aren't as good as hers. But you can't blame me for trying. What is magical about this dish is that it's a naturally vegan, gluten-free pancake with no need for binders at all. It was my favorite Korean food when I was growing up, and as an adult, I enjoy the kimchi-flecked version. But you can omit the kimchi if you're serving little ones.

MAKES 10 TO 12 PANCAKES

INGREDIENTS

For the pancakes

1 cup (100 g) mung beans or yellow split peas

2 cloves garlic

1 teaspoon toasted sesame oil

1 teaspoon sea salt

Avocado oil, for frying

1 bell pepper, thinly sliced

¼ onion, thinly sliced

2 scallions, sliced lengthwise, then quartered

For the dipping sauce

2 teaspoons toasted sesame oil

2 tablespoons tamari

2 tablespoons rice vinegar

2 scallions, minced

Optional

½ cup jarred kimchi, chopped

1 teaspoon toasted sesame seeds or gomasio

Dash of cayenne pepper or togarashi

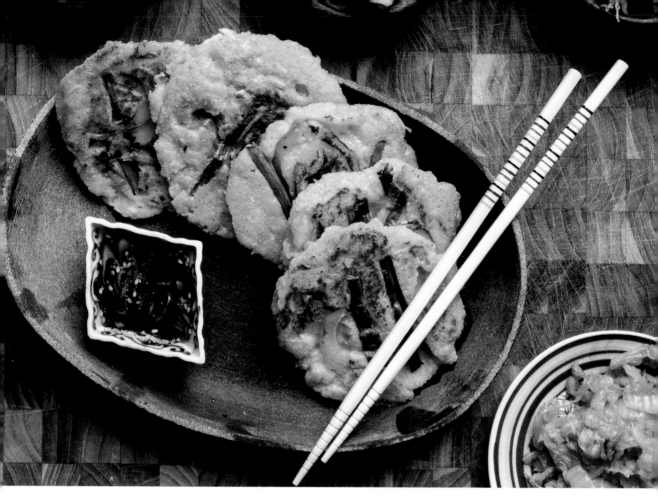

METHOD

Make the pancakes: Soak the beans in 3 cups (720 ml) water overnight or for at least 6 hours. Drain and rinse. Transfer the beans to a large food processor and add the garlic, kimchi (if using), sesame oil, salt, and ½ cup (120 ml) water. Blend to a pancake batter consistency.

Heat a nonstick skillet on medium-high heat and add 1 tablespoon of the avocado oil to the pan. Once the oil is sizzling, lower the heat to medium and place a ¼-cup (60-ml) scoop of batter in the pan. The pancake should start to sizzle. Add a couple of slices of the pepper, onion, and scallion

to the top of the pancake and pat down. Cook about 2 minutes and flip; cook the other side about 2 minutes. Continue to cook and flip the pancake about every 2 minutes, until it is crisp and brown on the outside. Transfer it to a dish towel–covered plate and let cool. Do the same with the remaining batter.

Make the dipping sauce: Whisk together the ingredients in a bowl and set aside.

Serve the pancakes with the dipping sauce.

CHICKPEA TUNA

This tuna salad might be the first time I ever got creative in the kitchen. I was about eleven or twelve and I wanted to make my own version of our household's lunchtime staple. We had some dried dill in the pantry, so I added it to the celery and onions that dad usually had with his tuna (which I agree is imperative). I sat solo in our breakfast room, eating my sublime creation on Melba toast, feeling pretty damn proud of myself. So this recipe is that—but grown up and plantified. I don't really eat tuna anymore—mercury and all—and for some inexplicable reason, chickpeas taste just like canned tuna.

MAKES 2 CUPS (340 G) TUNA

INGREDIENTS

1 (15½-ounce/439-g) can chickpeas, drained and rinsed, or 1½ cups cooked chickpeas

2 stalks celery, minced

1 shallot (3 ounces/85 g), minced,

¼ cup (30 g) capers, rinsed

¼ cup (2.5 g) chopped fresh dill

2 tablespoons chopped fresh parsley leaves

Juice of 1 lemon

1 tablespoon Dijon mustard

¼ cup (60 ml) olive oil

Sea salt

Freshly cracked black pepper

Optional

Dash of cayenne pepper

2 tablespoons Aquafaba Mayo or store-bought vegan mayo (optional; page 223)

Serve with

Crudités

Lettuce cups

Toasted pita or sourdough

METHOD

Combine drained chickpeas, celery, shallot, capers, dill, parsley, lemon, mustard, and oil in a bowl. Using a potato masher or fork, mash the chickpeas well until it forms a "tuna salad" consistency. Season with salt and pepper. For an "Italian-style" tuna salad, omit mayo. For a creamier consistency, add 2 tablespoons of mayo or more, depending on how creamy you like it. Squeeze in lemon juice and mix. Serve with crudités and cayenne, if using, atop a salad, or in pita pockets. You can store the tuna in an airtight container in the fridge for up to 5 days.

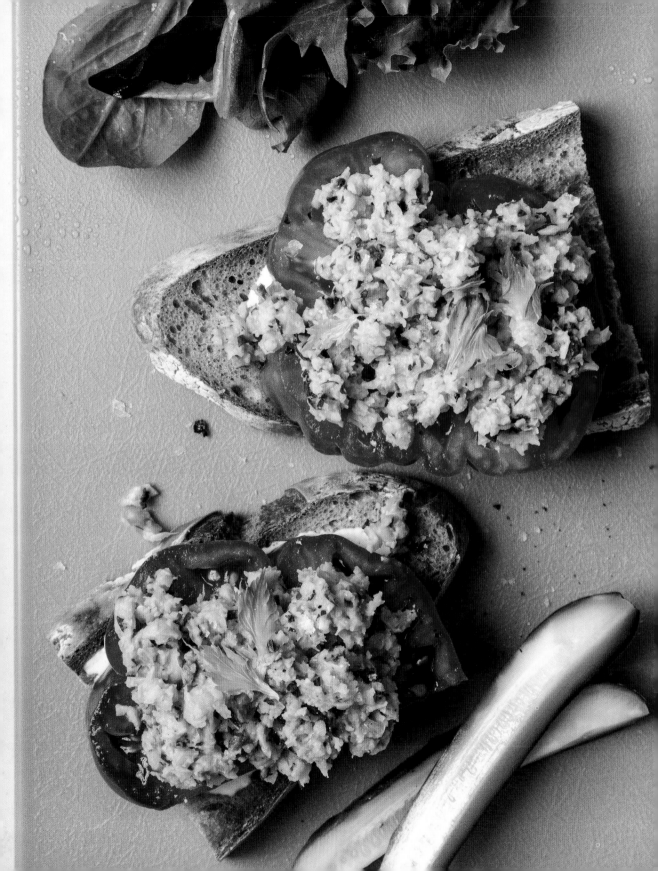

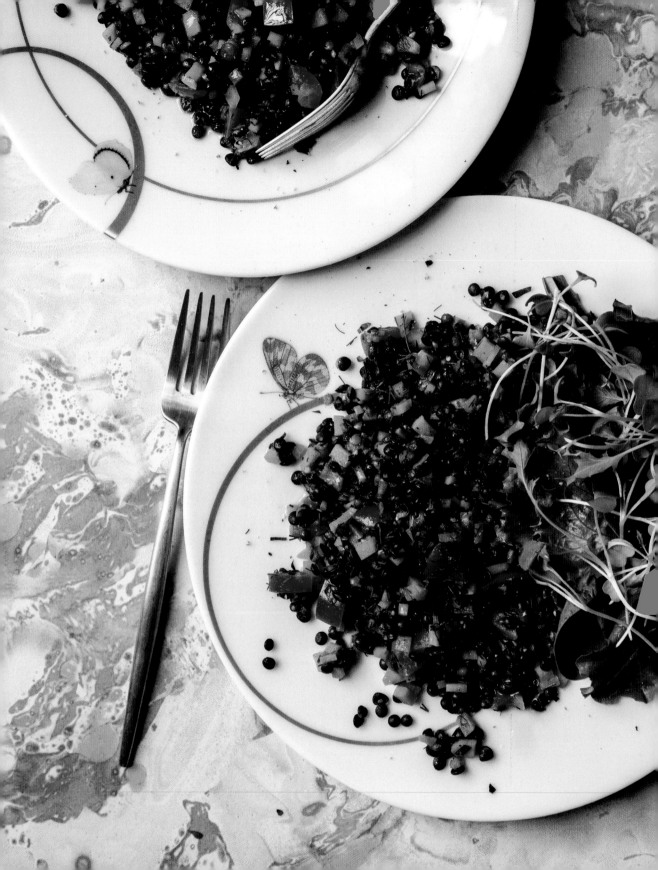

BELUGA LENTIL SALAD

There is something super refined about beluga lentils. Maybe because they're named after caviar. (Anything named after caviar must be a little fancy, I would think.) Slightly smaller than brown or green lentils and made to have a little more bite, they make the perfect vehicle for a bright vinaigrette. I love to keep this super-filling, fiber- and iron-rich dish in the fridge to add to salads or have as a snack with lettuce cups.

SERVES 2 TO 4

INGREDIENTS

For the lentils

1 cup (190 g) dried beluga lentils

1 tablespoon apple cider vinegar

½ teaspoon sea salt

1 sheet kombu

For the dressing

¼ cup (40 g) minced shallot

2 tablespoons apple cider vinegar

¼ cup (60 ml) olive oil

2 tablespoons Dijon mustard

2 tablespoons chopped fresh parsley

2 tablespoons chopped fresh dill

Sea salt

Freshly cracked black pepper

Garnish

1 large tomato, chopped

2 whole carrots, minced

For serving (optional)

Lettuce cups

METHOD

Make the lentils: In a bowl, add the vinegar and kombu to 2 cups (480 ml) water and soak the lentils overnight or for 6 hours. Soaking raw lentils in water, vinegar and kombu breaks down the outer layer of legumes and helps make them easier to digest and eliminate. Drain and fill a pot with water, add soaked lentils with salt and bring to a boil. Simmer on medium low heat, covered for 8 minutes. You want the lentils to be cooked but firm. Drain and rinse with cold water, and set aside in a serving bowl.

Make the dressing: In a small bowl, combine the shallot and vinegar and let sit for 10 to 15 minutes to slightly pickle. Add the oil, mustard, parsley, and dill and whisk together. Season with salt and pepper to taste. Pour the dressing over the cooked lentils and garnish with the tomato and carrots. Serve right away, or store in an airtight container in the fridge for up to 5 days.

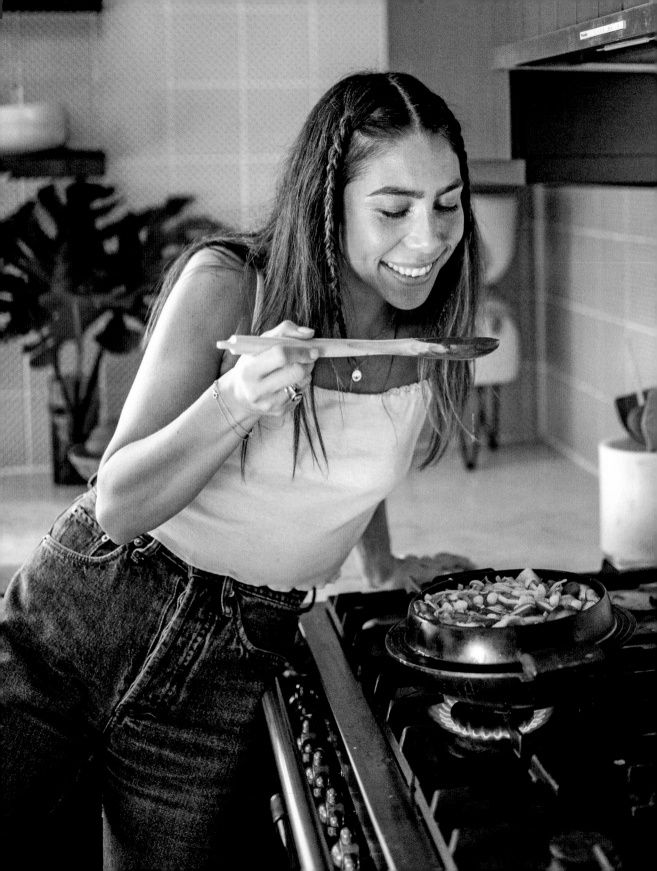

SOUPS

ANTI-INFLAMMATORY RED LENTIL STEW

A fter our New York City wedding, my husband Nick and I jetted to the Maldives, in the middle of the Indian Ocean, right off the coast of Sri Lanka. While we certainly did all the honeymoon-ish things (our firstborn, Jude, arrived ten months later), we also ate our weight in curries and South Indian stews, coconut rice, and rotis. It was here that I first tasted proper dal. This naturally vegan stew blew my mind. It's incredibly grounding and good for digestion (bye-bye, bloat), thanks to warming, anti-inflammatory spices, and perfect for those transitional fall-to-winter days, though sometimes I crave it with a dollop of cool, tangy coconut yogurt, even during the warmer months. I like to serve it with basmati rice and a simple salad of romaine, cilantro, and cucumber, with a cumin seed vinaigrette, to start.

SERVES 4 TO 6 PEOPLE

INGREDIENTS

For the lentil stew

2 tablespoons coconut oil or avocado oil

1 yellow onion, finely chopped

1-inch (2.5-cm) knob ginger, grated

3 cloves garlic, minced

1 teaspoon sea salt

¼ teaspoon freshly cracked black pepper

2 tablespoons garam masala or curry powder

1 (28-ounce/794-g) can crushed tomatoes

½ teaspoon ground cinnamon

½ teaspoon ground turmeric

1 cup (170 g) dried red lentils

Juice and zest of ½ lemon

4 tablespoons (22 g) roughly chopped cilantro leaves

For the cumin seed drizzle

¼ cup (60 ml) avocado oil

2 tablespoons cumin seeds

½ teaspoon sea salt

Optional

Dollop plain coconut yogurt

METHOD

Make the lentil stew: Rinse and drain the lentils until the water runs clear. Set aside.

In a large stockpot (with a capacity of 3 quarts/2.8 L, or more), heat the oil until melted. Add the onion, ginger, and garlic. Sauté on medium heat for about 3 minutes, or until fragrant. Be careful not to brown the onions; you want them to be translucent. Season with the salt and pepper and add the curry powder or garam masala, if using, cinnamon, and turmeric. Combine until the onions are well coated.

Add the lentils, tomatoes, and 4 to 6 cups (960 ml to 1.4 L) water to the pot and bring to a boil. Cover and simmer for 45 minutes to an hour, stirring occasionally.

Add the lemon juice and zest and taste, adding more salt and pepper, if desired. Turn off the heat.

Once the stew has cooled a bit, transfer half of it to a blender or food processor in batches and blend until creamy. Do not blend the other half of the stew; leave it chunky. Pour the blended soup back into the pot and combine. Stir in 2 tablespoons of the cilantro.

Make the cumin seed drizzle: In a small shallow pan, heat the oil for 2 to 3 minutes on medium heat. Add the cumin seeds and salt. Sauté on medium-low heat until fragrant and slightly browned, 1 to 2 minutes.

Serve the stew hot. Divide it among individual bowls and sprinkle with 2 tablespoons of the cilantro. Pour over the drizzle and top with the yogurt, if using.

Did you know red lentils are the easies to digest among the legume family and require the least amount of cooking time?

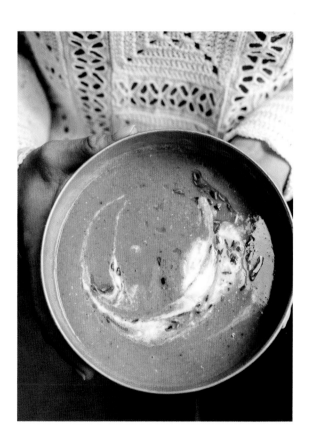

COCONUT PHO BOWLS

T his might be my favorite thing to make in the winter. Actually, in the summer too. It reminds me of the piping hot bowls Nick and I would get on the beach in Phuket. In fact, eating hot, steamy, soupy bowls can be quite cooling in the hotter months. The creamy, salty broth is so easy to make and, shockingly, you don't even need that much time. Fifteen minutes for a fragrant multilayered broth? You bet. It's also hard to mess up if you have the right aromatics. You can add pretty much any vegetables you have on hand and it'll still be great. What makes this soup, though, are the fresh and bright herbs and the crunchy, spicy fixings. And don't forget the lime wedge for extra alkalinity.

MAKES 4 TO 5 BOWLS

INGREDIENTS

2 tablespoons coconut oil

2 cloves garlic, smashed and minced

1 large yellow onion, minced

1-inch (2.5-cm) knob turmeric, or ½ teaspoon dried

1½- to 2-inch (4- to 5-cm) knob ginger, grated

1 teaspoon sea salt

3 scallions, halved

2 cups (115 g) cooked vermicelli

1 (13½-ounce/398-ml) can full-fat unsweetened coconut milk

1 cup (75 g) napa cabbage, thinly sliced

3 carrots, peeled and shaved

1 red bell pepper, cored and thinly sliced

1 cup (96 g) shiitake mushrooms caps, sliced

2 cups (142 g) broccoli florets and stems, roughly chopped

1 tablespoon coconut sugar

Juice and zest of 1 lime

2 tablespoons tamari sauce

1 zucchini, shaved into "noodles" with a serrated vegetable peeler or thinly sliced into long strips

Optional

¼ cup (60 ml) Vegan Fish Sauce (page 219)

Garnish

½ cup fresh mint leaves

½ cup fresh cilantro leaves

½ cup lightly packed fresh basil leaves

¼ cup roasted peanuts, crushed or roughly chopped

1 lime, quartered

Thinly sliced Bird's Eye Chili, or, red chili flakes, or chili oil

½ cup raw bean sprouts

METHOD

In a 3-quart (2.8-L) stockpot, heat the coconut oil. When it has melted, add the garlic, onion, turmeric, and ginger and sauté on medium low for 2 minutes, until fragrant, being careful not to brown. Add 6 cups (1.4 L) water, the fish sauce, if using, and the scallions. Season with salt. Bring to a boil, then simmer for 15 minutes or up to an hour, depending on how much time you have.

While the broth is simmering, in a pot of boiled water, off heat, hydrate the vermicelli, loosening the strands for 3 to 4 minutes. Drain and rinse with cold water. Separate the strands with your hands. If you're not using the noodles right away, you can add 1 tablespoon avocado oil and massage them to prevent clumping.

Once the broth has finished simmering, turn off the heat and add the milk. Combine well. Bring to a low simmer and add the cabbage, carrots, bell pepper, mushrooms, and broccoli. Simmer for 3 to 5 minutes, until the vegetables are tender but still bright and al dente. Add the sugar, lime juice and zest, and tamari and salt to taste.

In 4 or 5 deep soup bowls, nestle ½ cup cooked noodles and ¼ cup zucchini noodles then ladle 1 to 2 cups vegetables and broth over the noodles. Garnish with mint, cilantro, and basil and crushed peanuts. Add a lime wedge, bean sprouts, and the chili flakes or chili oil. Serve immediately.

When sourcing canned coconut milks, I look for organic, unsweetened, and brands that do not use any gums or additives as binders.

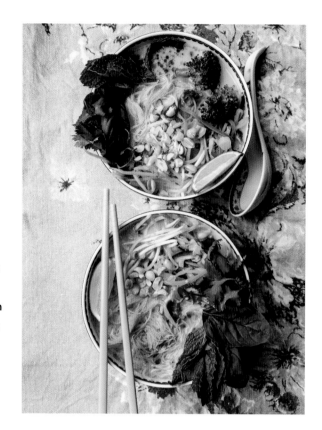

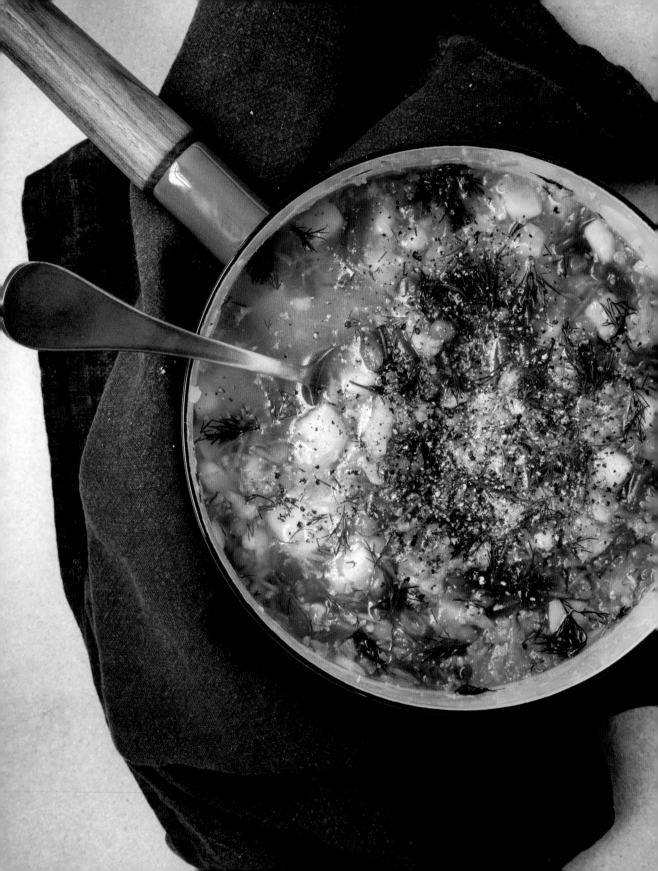

BABUSHKA SOUP

T his recipe was created for my husband, who was born in the former USSR. When we were dating, we used to spend late nights at Webster Hall at a Ukrainian diner in the East Village called Veselka. He would get pierogi and kasha and I would get this dilled vegetable soup. It's the first non-pureed recipe I would make for our son, Jude, and in the winters, we have a big batch in the fridge at all times.

SERVES 4 TO 6

INGREDIENTS

2 tablespoons grass-fed butter or ghee (could use vegan butter or avocado oil to make vegan)

1 large yellow onion, peeled and minced

1½ teaspoons sea salt

3 large carrots, peeled and shredded

1½ cups (170 g) green beans, snipped and chopped

1 head cauliflower (6 ounces /170 g), cored and roughly chopped

2 russet potatoes, peeled and chopped into ⅓-inch cubes

1 cup (135 g) frozen peas, thawed

Zest of 1 lemon

Juice of ½ lemon

Freshly cracked black pepper

2 to 3 tablespoons freshly chopped dill, or more (I like this soup really dill-y.)

METHOD

In a large stockpot (with a capacity of about 5½ quarts/ 1.3 L), heat the butter/ghee or oil. When the butter has melted, add the onion and sauté on medium-low heat until fragrant and translucent but not brown, about 2½ minutes, stirring occasionally. Season with ½ teaspoon of the salt. Add the chopped carrots, beans, cauliflower, and potatoes. Add 6 cups (1.4 L) water and bring to a boil, then simmer, covered, for 30 to 40 minutes. At 30 minutes, add the peas and add more salt if needed.

Once the soup is done, add the lemon zest, juice, and black pepper. Off heat, stir in the chopped dill. Serve immediately.

What makes this soup is shredding the carrots on the small hole side of a box grater. The carrots will emulsify into the broth, leaving a silky, slightly sweet earthy flavor and texture.

TOMATO COCONUT MILK BISQUE

There is something so retro about tomato soup. Maybe it's because of the throwback canned versions or the kind they serve at the diner with grilled cheese. This version is as creamy as the one you remember, with a slight southeast Asian twist thanks to the coconut and ginger.

MAKES 8 CUPS (2 L) SOUP

INGREDIENTS

2 tablespoons coconut oil

2 to 3 cloves garlic, minced

2-inch (5-cm) knob ginger, peeled and grated

1 large yellow onion, peeled and chopped

1 large red bell pepper, peeled and chopped

1 teaspoon sea salt

Freshly cracked black pepper

1 (28-ounce/794-g) can crushed San Marzano tomatoes

2 (13½-ounce/398-ml) cans unsweetened coconut milk

METHOD

In a 3¼-quart pot, heat the oil until melted. Add the garlic, ginger, and onion and sauté on medium-high heat until fragrant and translucent, 3 to 4 minutes. Add the red pepper and sauté for 3 to 5 minutes more, until pepper is tender. Season with ½ teaspoon of the salt and with black pepper to taste. Add the tomatoes and bring to a boil. Simmer, covered, for 20 minutes. Turn off the heat and let cool.

Transfer the tomato mixture to a blender or use an immersion blender and blend for 1 to 2 minutes, until super creamy. Transfer the mixture back to the pot and heat on low. Pour in the milk and gently stir. Simmer for another 5 minutes more, if you like, and season with the remaining ½ teaspoon salt and freshly cracked pepper, as needed.

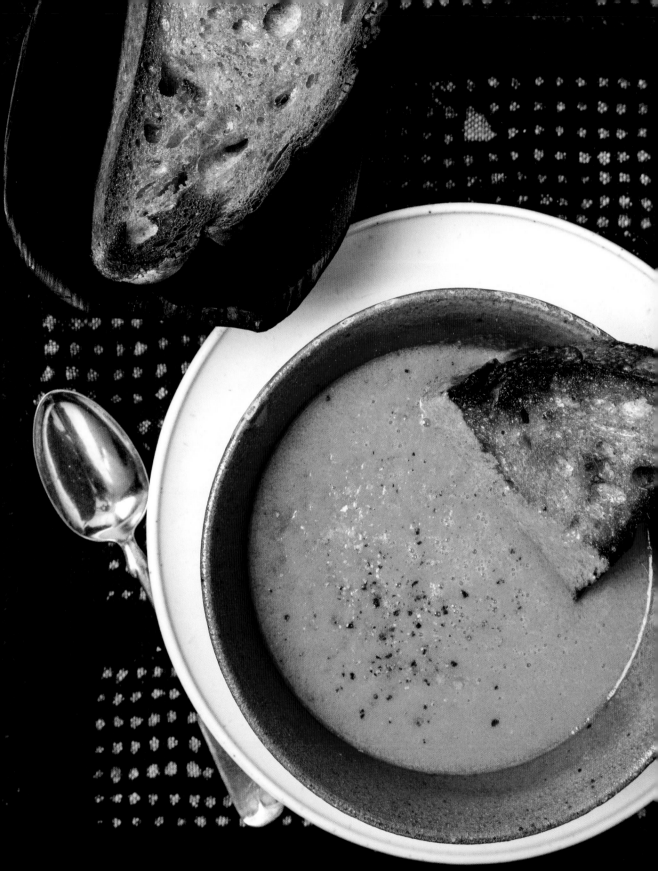

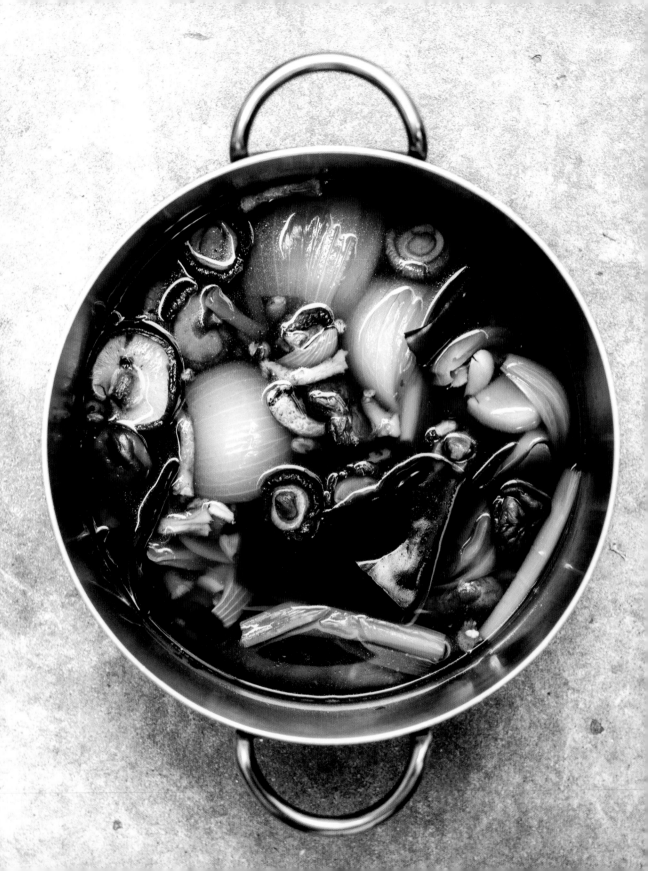

VEGAN DASHI BROTH

The universal broth base has so many purposes and can serve as the base of any Asian soup dish or lend an earthy, umami flavor to any soup. Rich in minerals thanks to the kombu and dulse, it's almost like a vegan bone broth and can be enjoyed sipped through a mug as a healing simple broth. It is also a great base for any of the noodle soups or Asian stews in this book.

MAKES 6 CUPS (1.4 L) BROTH

INGREDIENTS

3 strips kombu (1¼ ounces/35 g)

1 cup (35 g) dried shiitake mushrooms or any dried mushrooms

2 cups (140 g) fresh mushroom stems

4 large cloves garlic

2½-inch (6-cm) knob ginger, peeled

¼ cup (11 g) dulse seaweed

1 medium onion

2 scallions

METHOD

In a saucepan, combine all the ingredients with 6 cups (1.4 L) water, bring to a boil, and then simmer for at least 30 minutes. Let cool, then drain and discard solids. Transfer the broth to an airtight container. It will keep in the fridge for up to a week, or you can freeze it for several weeks.

You can find kombu, dulse seaweed and dried shiitake mushrooms at most health food shops or Asian markets.

SEA'S HEARTY MISO STEW

As the name suggests, this is our daughter Sea's favorite soup. Similar to a traditional miso soup, it's packed with veggies and mineral-rich seaweed, making it a nourishing, grounding meal in and of itself.

SERVES 4 TO 6

INGREDIENTS

6 cups (1.4 L) water, Vegan Dashi (page 157), or vegetable broth

2 tablespoons red or white miso paste (if using water, use 3 tablespoons miso)

½ sweet or yellow onion, thinly sliced

1 clove garlic, minced

2-inch (5-cm) knob ginger, peeled, or 1 teaspoon grated ginger

1 tablespoon tamari (if using water)

½ cup (75 g) frozen edamame beans, shelled and thawed

2 cups (155 g) shiitake mushroom caps, thinly sliced

3 medium carrots, shredded (½ cup/105g)

2 cups (150 g) shredded napa cabbage

2 tablespoons rice vinegar

½ cup (75 g) hydrated wakame seaweed

½ cup (75 g) hydrated arame seaweed, cut into bite-size pieces

Garnish (optional)

Sliced scallions

Toasted sesame seeds

Optional

Rice, udon, or soba noodles, cooked as directed on box

METHOD

In a large stockpot, combine the water or broth, miso, and onion and bring to a boil. Add the garlic, ginger, and tamari, if using, and simmer for 5 minutes. Add the edamame and shiitake and simmer for 5 minutes more. Add the carrots. Turn off the heat and add the cabbage and seaweed. Let sit for a couple of minutes for the cabbage to soften. If using, add 1 handful of noodles to bowls and ladle broth over. Serve in bowls garnished with sliced scallions and sesame seeds, if using.

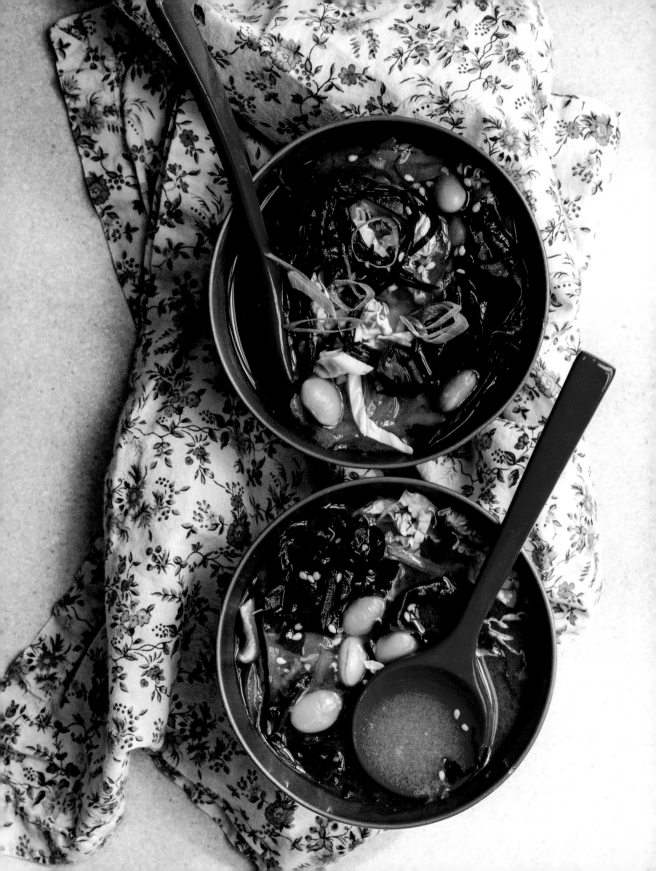

CAULIFLOWER BISQUE

This is one of the first recipes I ever posted on my website, bonberi.com. It's one of the simplest, but also delicious and cleansing and barely requires any thought. I consider it a starter recipe for the Body Harmony life and a great basic soup to keep in the fridge on those transitional fall-to-winter days.

SERVES 4 TO 6

INGREDIENTS

2 tablespoons avocado oil

4 cloves garlic, minced (2 tablespoons)

1 yellow onion, chopped (2½ cups/ 400 g)

½ teaspoon salt

Freshly cracked black pepper

1 medium head cauliflower cut into florets and stems (7 cups/840 g)

¼ cup (60 ml) olive oil

Juice and zest of 1 lemon

METHOD

In a large pot, heat the avocado oil over medium-high heat. Add the garlic, onion, salt, and pepper to taste, and saute for 3 to 4 minutes until fragrant and the onion begins to soften. Add the cauliflower and 6 cups (1.4 L) water and simmer for 20 minutes. Let cool.

Transfer to a food processor or blender and blend for 1 minute, slowly adding the oil. Return to the pot and add the lemon juice and zest and more salt and pepper to taste. Serve hot.

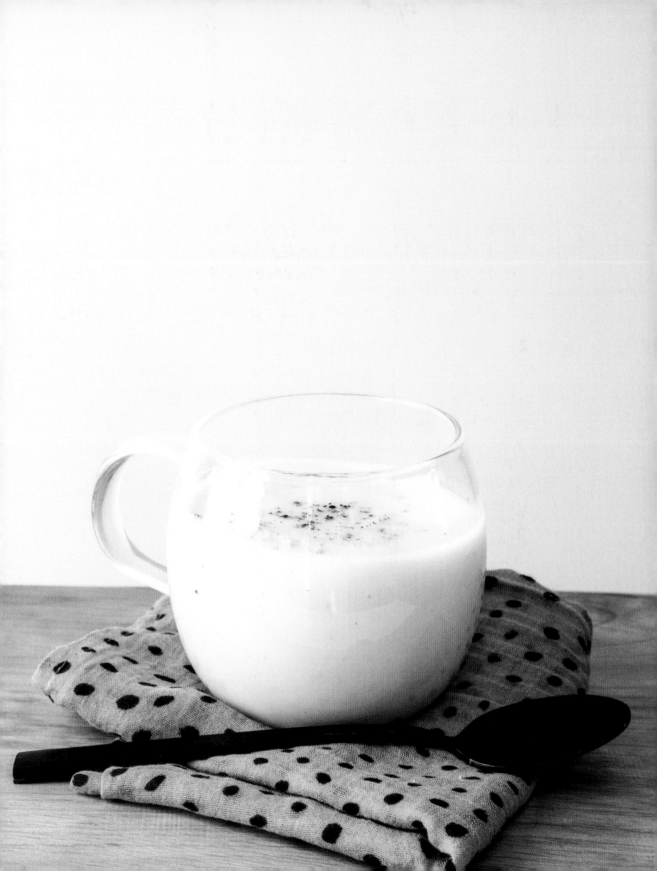

GAZPACHO

always thought I disliked gazpacho—you know, the chunky kind that feels like a salad smoothie gone wrong. But after many summers in Ibiza, I've fallen in love with the classic Balearic version of this dish. It's perfectly smooth and velvety, slightly sweet and incredibly soothing on a hot summer's eve.

SERVES 2 TO 4

INGREDIENTS

4 to 5 ripe large tomatoes, roughly chopped (3 pounds/1360 g)

½ red bell pepper, cored and roughly chopped (2 ounces/56 g)

1 peeled cucumber, halved (11¾ ounces/335 g)

¼ yellow or white onion (2½ ounces/68 g)

1 tablespoon apple cider vinegar

¼ cup of olive oil (2 ounces/60 ml)

1 clove garlic

Sea salt and pepper to taste

Garnish

2 tablespoons diced bell pepper

2 tablespoons diced cucumber

METHOD

Add all the ingredients to a blender and blend until smooth. Garnish with diced pepper and cucumbers. Chill for at least 1 hour.

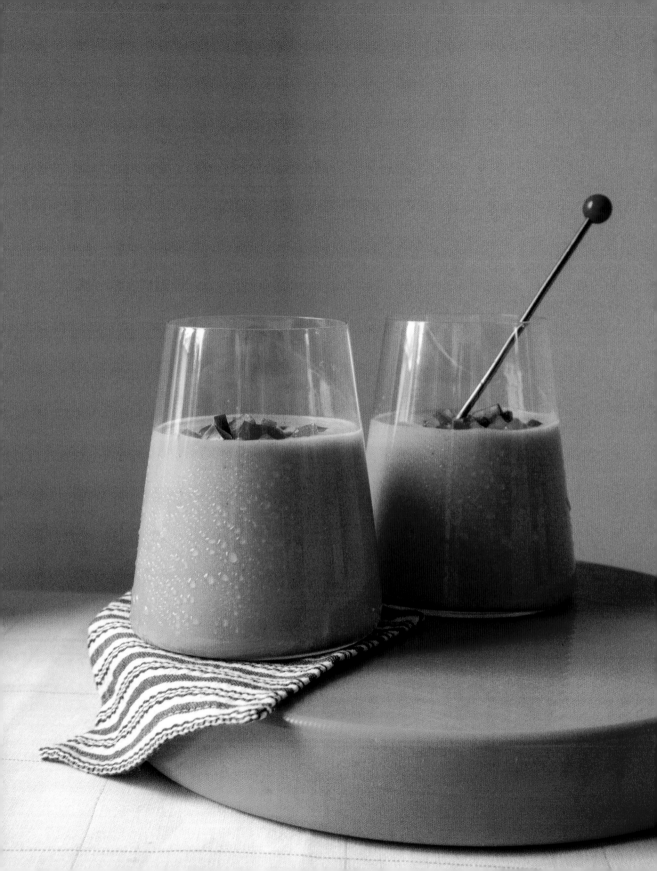

CARROT GINGER SOUP

On weeks when I want a reboot, I always make this soup. Packed with vitamin C and anti-inflammatory ginger, it's amazing for immune support and yet so comforting. The cilantro drizzle gives it a little something, but you can omit the ginger and cilantro for a kiddo- and even post-six-month-old-baby-friendly option.

SERVES 4 TO 6

INGREDIENTS

2 tablespoons avocado oil

1 large chopped onion, or 3 cups (390 g) chopped onion

2-inch knob ginger, grated, or 2½ teaspoons grated ginger

1 clove garlic, grated

5 cups (680 g) carrots, chopped

1 teaspoon ground coriander

1 teaspoon sea salt (or more, as needed)

1 (13½-ounce/398-ml) can coconut milk

Zest of 1 lemon

Freshly cracked black pepper

1 tablespoon Cilantro Drizzle (recipe follows)

CILANTRO DRIZZLE

MAKES ⅔ CUP (165 ML) DRIZZLE

INGREDIENTS

1 bunch cilantro

3 to 4 cloves garlic

1 teaspoon grated ginger

½ cup (120 ml) olive oil

1 tablespoon maple syrup

2 tablespoons fresh lemon juice

1 jalapeño chile, seeded

Sea salt

Freshy cracked black pepper

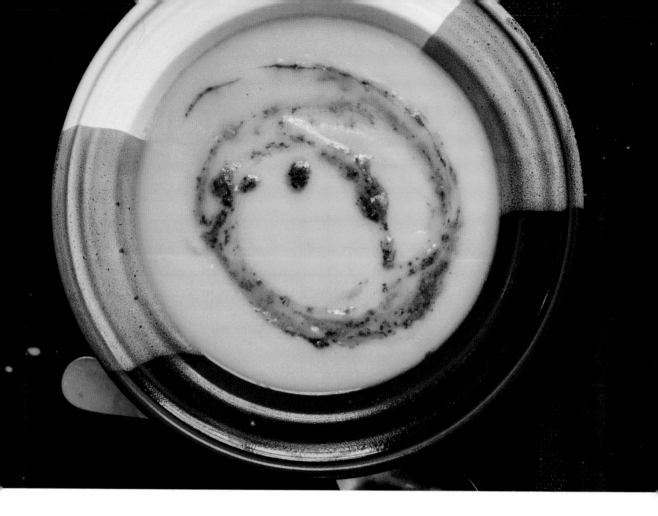

METHOD

In a large pot over medium heat, heat the oil. Add the onion, ginger, and garlic and sauté for 3 to 4 minutes, until fragrant and translucent. Reduce heat to low and add the carrots and coriander. Sauté for 2 to 3 minutes more. Add 4 to 5 cups (960 ml to 1.3 L) water and the salt. Bring to a boil, then reduce the heat and simmer for 35 minutes, or until the carrots are tender. Cool and transfer to a blender and blend for 1 minute, until smooth. Transfer back to the pot and bring to a low simmer. Add the milk and lemon zest and season with more salt and pepper, if needed.

To make the cilantro drizzle: In a blender, blend the cilantro, garlic, ginger, oil, syrup, lemon juice, and jalapeño until smooth and bright. Season with salt and pepper to taste.

Transfer the carrot mixture to serving bowls and spoon the drizzle on top. You can omit the drizzle if you're serving kids.

LEAN GREEN SOUP

W hen I'm looking to ground down and re-center myself, this is one of the first things I make to keep in my fridge for the week. Green soups can be, well, disenchanting. But this version is packed with flavor and it's creamy, thanks to the coconut, which makes it almost decadent. You could blend it for a classic "detox" soup, but I sometimes like to leave mine whole for a heartier stew.

SERVES 4 TO 6

INGREDIENTS

2 tablespoons coconut oil

2 cloves garlic, minced

1 onion, chopped

2 teaspoons grated ginger

2 cups (178 g) roughly chopped celery

1 bunch broccoli, stems and florets, chopped, or 6 cups (531 g) chopped

1 zucchini (7½ ounces/215 g), chopped

1 fennel bulb (10 ounces/280 g), chopped

½ teaspoon ground coriander

Sea salt

Freshly cracked black pepper

2 cups (67 g) destemmed and roughly chopped kale

2 cups (85 g) roughly chopped spinach

1 (13½-ounce/398-ml) can simple coconut milk

Juice and zest of 1 lime

Garnish

Fresh cilantro

Lime wedges

METHOD

In a large pot, heat the oil. Add the garlic, onion, 1 teaspoon of the ginger, and celery and sauté until fragrant, 3 to 5 minutes. Add the broccoli, zucchini, fennel, and coriander. Cover with water and bring to a boil. Reduce heat and simmer, covered, for about 7 minutes.

Season with sea salt and pepper to taste. You want the greens to be cooked but still bright. Add the kale and spinach and cover, allowing the greens to wilt, about 2 minutes. Remove from the heat and let cool. It's your choice whether to blend the soup in batches or keep it chunky. If blending, blend the vegetable mixture first before adding the milk, lime juice and zest, and the remaining 1 teaspoon ginger. Transfer the soup to a serving bowl and garnish with cilantro and lime wedges.

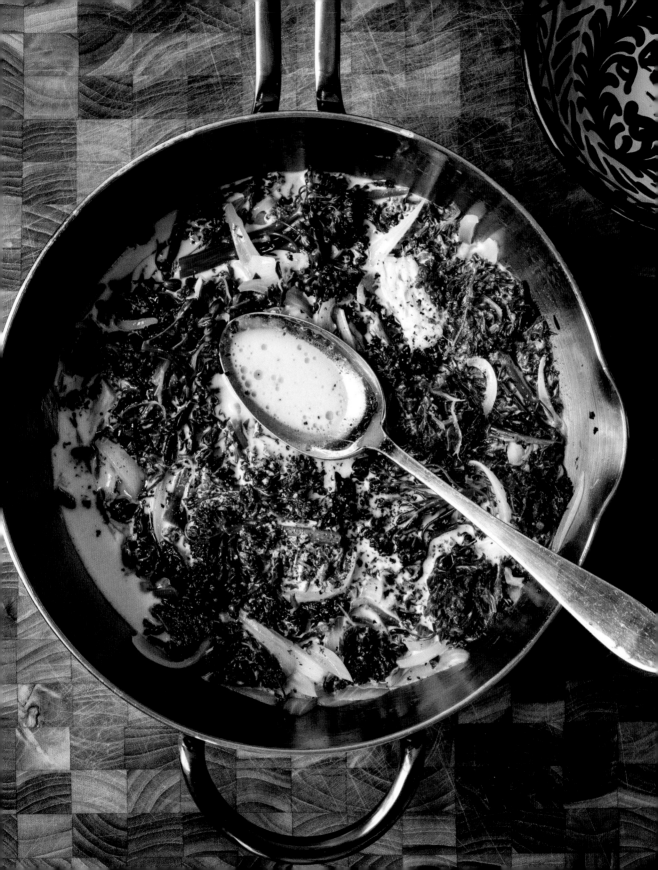

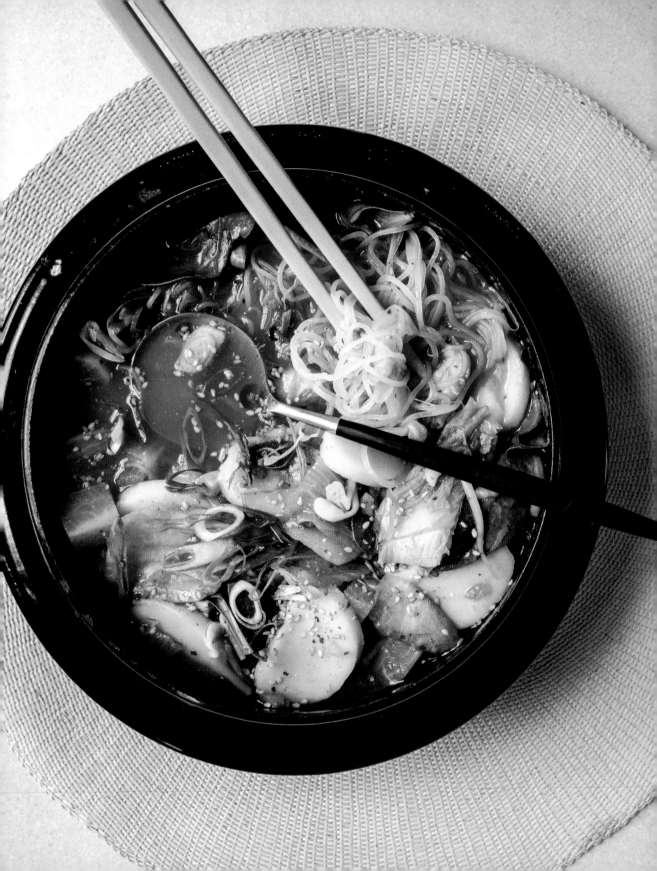

LUNAR NEW YEAR RICE CAKE SOUP

Some people have matzo ball soup, and some chicken noodle; growing up, I had this. A sometimes spicy, simmering broth served literally boiling hot, this vat of goodness can cure anything you've got, I'm convinced. In Korea, it's typically served on the New Year for good luck, but you can have it anytime for a solid soul soothing. You can omit the kimchi if you don't want your broth too spicy. You can find Korean rice cakes in the frozen section in any Asian market or online.

SERVES 4 TO 6

INGREDIENTS

5 cups (1.2 L) Vegan Dashi Broth (page 157) or water

1 tablespoon white or red miso paste

1 daikon radish, peeled and chopped

2 scallions, thinly sliced

1 white onion, peeled and chopped

6 cloves garlic, minced

3 stalks celery, chopped

2-inch knob ginger, grated

2 tablespoons tamari

1 teaspon toasted sesame oil

1 teaspoon sea salt

2 cups (245 g) frozen rice cakes, defrosted

1 cup (90 g) mung bean sprouts

3 cups (170 g) shiitake mushrooms

2 cups (100 g) bunapi or straw mushrooms

2 cups (85 g) packed spinach

2 cups (300 g) cooked mung bean or kelp noodles

Optional (to make spicy)

1 (16-ounce) jar kimchi, chopped

Garnish

1 sheet nori, cut into strips

METHOD

In a large pot, combine the broth, miso paste, radish, scallions, onion, garlic, celery, ginger tamari, sesame oil, and salt and bring to a boil. Reduce to a strong simmer/low bowl, covered, for 10 to 15 minutes. Add defrosted rice cakes, bean sprouts, shiitakes, bunapis or straw mushrooms, and kimchi (if using). Simmer, covered, for another 10 to 15 minutes until rice cakes are soft, continuing to stir to make sure the rice cakes don't stick to the bottom of the pot. Remove the lid from the pot once the veggies are cooked and stir in the spinach and noodles. Continue on a low boil for 2 minutes more. Serve the broth boiling hot in stone bowls or soup bowls. Top with the nori.

CHICKPEA AND KALE COCONUT CURRY

I love this meal for a hearty weeknight dinner. The coconut milk feels so indulgent, like a warm hug. It's one pan, so it's not fussy at all, and it's incredibly filling. I love to serve it with grain-free roti or a bowl of fluffy basmati rice.

SERVES 2 TO 4

INGREDIENTS

2 teaspoons garam masala or curry powder

½ teaspoon ground turmeric

2 teaspoons cumin seeds

Freshly cracked black pepper

2 tablespoons coconut oil

1 large onion, minced, or 2 cups (305 g) minced onion

2-inch (5-cm) knob ginger (1 ounce/28 g), or 2 teaspoons grated

2 cloves garlic, minced

1 large tomato, or 1 cup (55 g) chopped

1 teaspoon sea salt

Dash of cayenne pepper

1½ cups cooked chickpeas, or 1 (15½-ounce/439-g) can chickpeas, drained and rinsed

1 bunch kale, chopped

1 teaspoon coconut sugar

1 (13½-ounce/398-ml) can simple coconut milk

½ cup (107 g) shredded unsweetened coconut

Juice of ½ lemon

Garnish

¼ cup (25 g) toasted shredded coconut

Fresh cilantro

METHOD

In a large pot, combine the garam masala, turmeric, cumin seeds, and freshly cracked black pepper to taste and lightly toast on medium-high heat for 1 minute. Add the oil, onion, ginger, garlic, tomato, salt, and cayenne. Lower the heat to medium and sauté for 5 minutes. Add the chickpeas, kale, and sugar and combine well. Add ¾ cup (180 ml) water and the milk, bring to a boil, and then simmer for 10 minutes. At 7 minutes, stir in the coconut and lemon juice.

While the curry is cooking, lightly toast the coconut for garnish until lightly browned. Transfer the coconut curry to bowls and top with the toasted coconut and cilantro. Serve with gluten-free tortillas, pita, or basmati rice.

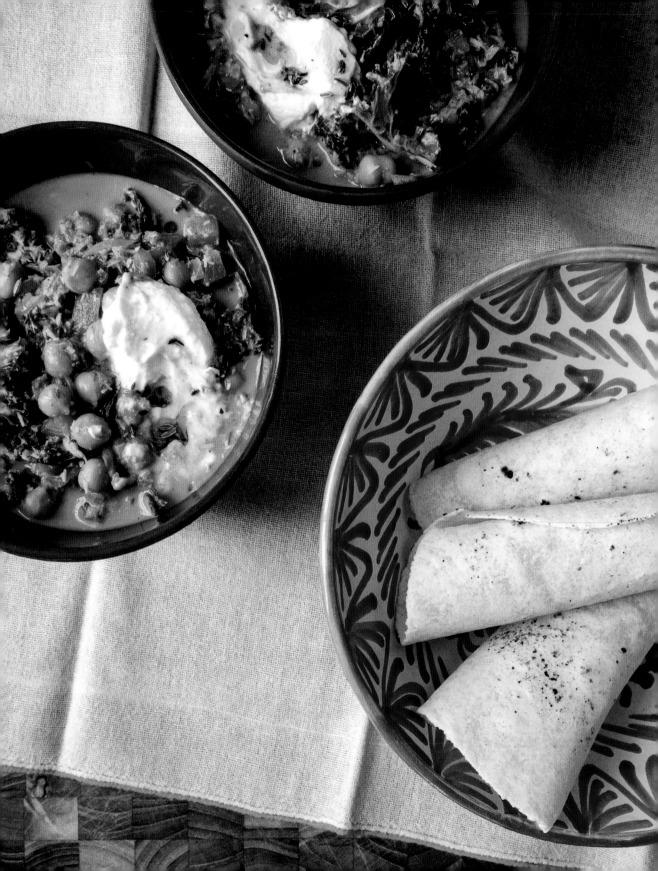

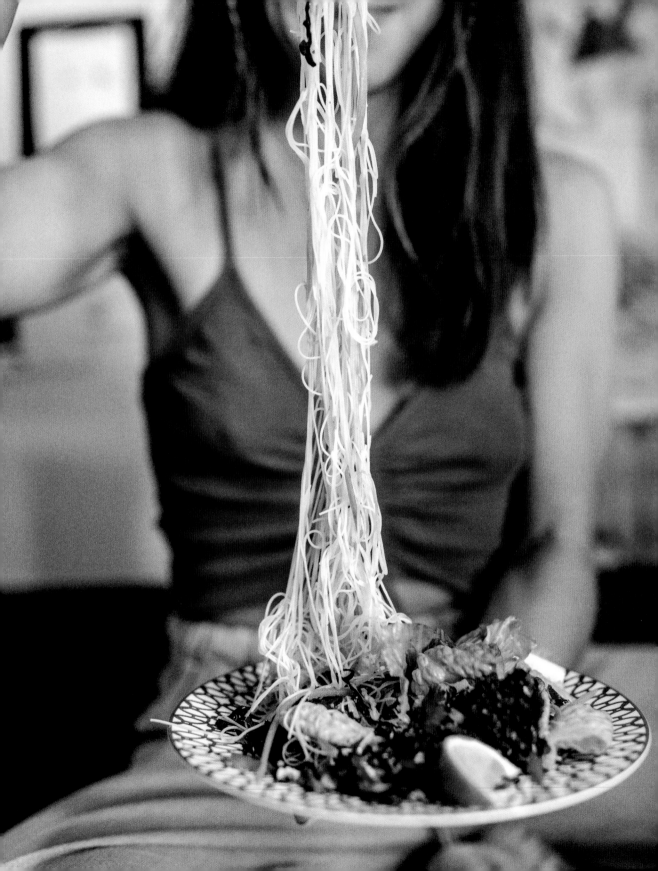

GRAINS

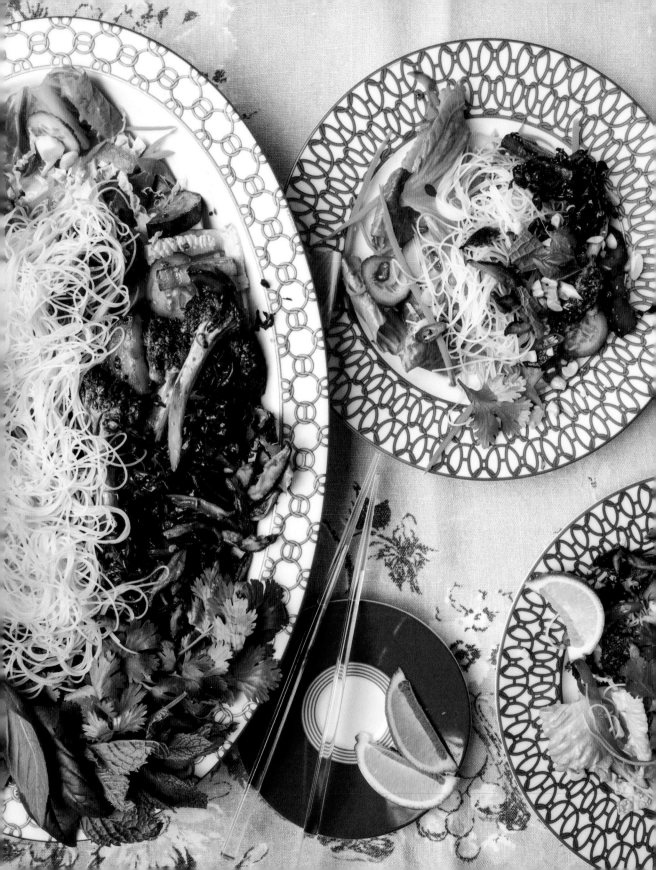

VIETNAMESE VERMICELLI NOODLE SALAD

would have a version of this salad for dinner weekly while I was at college in Boston, where Vietnamese dives abounded, and I never got over the flavors. The mint! The basil! The cilantro! Oh, this trifecta of herbs is unparalleled. There's something about the noodles, warm vegetables, and crunchy greens that really satisfies me on multiple levels. I also love that the salad doesn't require an oil-based dressing, which makes it one of the most cleansing dishes in the book. Don't skimp on the herbs and chile here—they make the dish!

SERVES 4 GENEROUSLY

INGREDIENTS

For the sautéed vegetables

2 tablespoons coconut oil, avocado oil, or a neutral oil

1 clove garlic, minced

1 teaspoon grated ginger

1 cup (215 g) broccoli florets

1 small zucchini, cut into ½-inch (12-mm) half-moons

1 cup (208 g) shiitake mushroom caps, thinly sliced

1 cup (210 g) bean sprouts

½ cup (75 g) frozen green peas, thawed

2 tablespoons tamari

1 tablespoon rice vinegar

Salt

Freshly cracked black pepper

For the raw vegetables

1 red bell pepper, cored and thinly sliced

1 head romaine, thinly sliced

1 cup (65 g) thinly sliced kale

1 cup (210 g) thinly sliced napa cabbage

1 large cucumber, peeled and sliced, or 2 Persian cucumbers, thinly sliced

2 large carrots, peeled and cut into matchsticks

For the noodles

2 cups (100 g) cooked rice vermicelli noodles, prepared according to package instructions

Garnish

1 jalapeño chile or red chile, deseeded and sliced

½ cup (12 g) fresh mint leaves, chopped

½ cup (9 g) fresh cilantro leaves, chopped

½ cup (10 g) fresh basil leaves, chopped

½ cup (125 g) crushed peanuts

½ cup (100 ml) Vietnamese Nuoc Cham Dressing (opposite)

1 lime, quartered

METHOD

Prepare the sautéed vegetables: In a shallow pan, melt the coconut oil. Add the garlic and ginger and sauté on low heat until fragrant, about 1 minute. Add the broccoli, zucchini, mushrooms, sprouts, peas, tamari, and vinegar and sauté until lightly browned, about 10 minutes. If the veggies are sticking to the pan, add a little water. Season with salt and pepper to taste. Remove from the heat and let cool.

Assemble the salad: In a large serving bowl or on a large serving platter, layer all the raw vegetables. Add the noodles and cooked vegetables. Top with the jalapeño, mint, cilantro, basil, and peanuts. Pour the dressing over the salad and serve immediately, with the lime wedges.

VIETNAMESE NUOC CHAM DRESSING

I love this dressing because it's oil-free yet packed with flavor. Salty, sour, spicy, and sweet, it hits all the notes. You could totally sub tamari for the fish sauce, but if you want to go the extra authenticity mile, use the sauce.

MAKES 1 CUP (240 ML) DRESSING

INGREDIENTS

1 teaspoon grated ginger

1 clove garlic, grated

2 tablespoons maple syrup or honey

¼ cup (60 ml) rice vinegar

1 tablespoon toasted sesame oil

2 tablespoons tamari

¼ cup (60 ml) Vegan Fish Sauce (page 219), or 2 more tablespoons tamari

1 tablespoon coconut sugar

½ jalapeño chile or Thai bird's eye chile, seeded and thinly sliced

Juice and zest of 1 lime

Sea salt

Freshly cracked pepper

METHOD

In a medium bowl, whisk the ginger, garlic, syrup, vinegar, oil, tamari, fish sauce, sugar, jalapeño, lime juice and zest, and ⅓ cup (75 ml) water. Season with salt and pepper to taste. The dressing will keep in the fridge in an airtight container for up to a week.

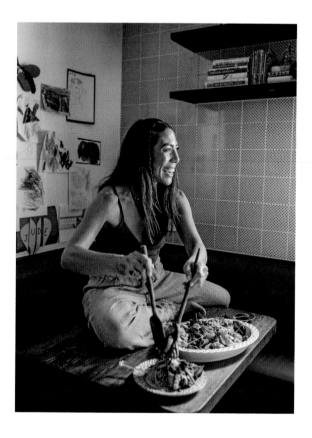

SOBA NOODLE SALAD

I have fond memories of eating soba when I was young. Some afternoons after school, my mom would take my brother and me to a Japanese supermarket complex in New Jersey. After she went grocery shopping and my brother and I stocked up on Super Mario and Sanrio paraphernalia, we would go to the food court and pick one of the delicacies displayed as plastic models for an afternoon snack. I always went for the cold soba that came with a delicate dipping sauce that I would plunge the noodles into and slurp happily, leaving brown spots all over the counter. This is my ode to that dish, packed with veggies for good measure.

SERVES 2

INGREDIENTS

For 2 Bowls

2 cups (225 g) cooked soba noodles, chilled (opposite)

2 cups (60 g) packed baby spinach

2 Persian cucumbers (7 ounces/200 g), thinly sliced

½ cup (30 g) shredded napa cabbage

Optional

Sliced avocado

Chopped kimchi

Steamed broccoli florets

Shiso leaves

For the dressing

1 cup (240 ml) Tamari Vinaigrette (page 214)

METHOD

In individual-size bowls, combine all the salad ingredients. Garnish with your choice of the avocado, kimchi, broccoli, and shiso. Pour the dressing over the salad and serve! You can also serve the dressing separately, in a large bowl, for dipping the noodles and vegetables.

BASIC SOBA NOODLES

Soba noodles are tricky to cook, especially when they are 100 percent buckwheat (many varieties are wheat and white flour blends). But, after many tries, I've perfected the job. Just follow step by step.

SERVES 2 TO 4

INGREDIENTS

8 ounces (225 g) 100% buckwheat soba noodles

½ cup (120 ml) ice cubes

1 teaspoon avocado oil or toasted sesame oil (see Note)

METHOD

Boil 6 cups (1.4 L) unsalted water. Add the noodles and, on medium-high heat, bring to a rolling boil. With a wooden spoon, begin to gently break apart the noodles, preventing them from clumping together. As the noodles cook, stay vigilant, continuing to gently break apart the noodles while taking care not to break them. After 7 to 8 minutes, transfer the pot to the sink and rinse with cold water. Gently break apart the noodles, rubbing them between your fingers under the cold water. The water should turn from murky to clear. Once you have removed all the starch, place the ice cubes in the bowl and set it aside until the noodles are needed.

Note: If you are cooking the noodles to use later, add the oil and massage the noodles gently to prevent them from clumping.

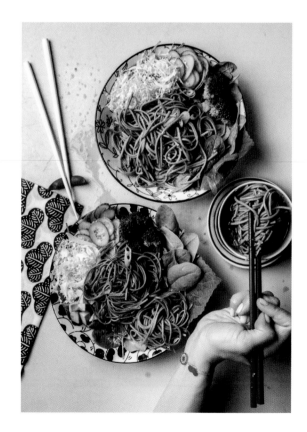

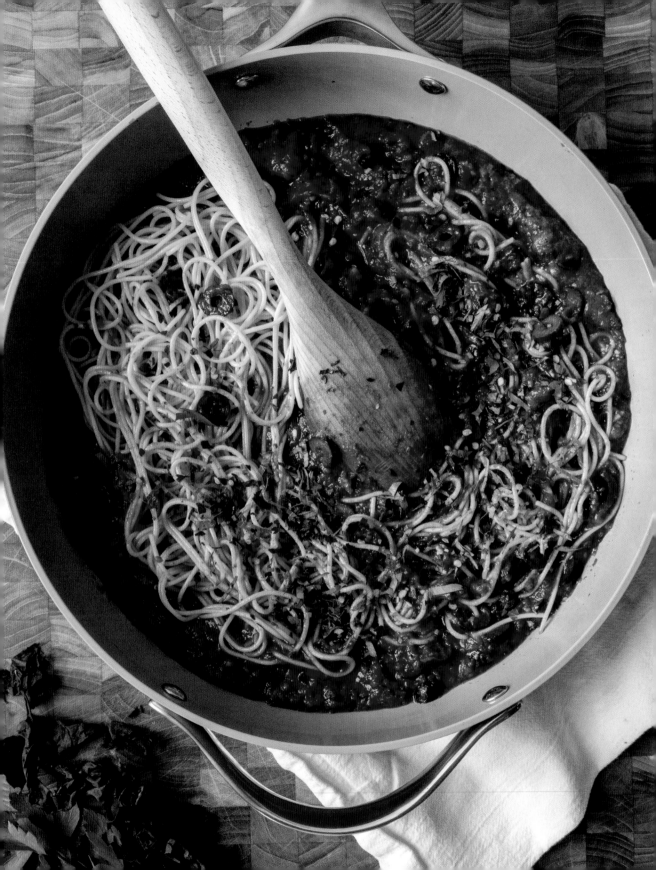

DULSE PUTTANESCA

love pasta. Who doesn't, right? There could probably be plenty more pasta dishes in this book, but I chose to include my top three that I make on the regular. This one is a crowd pleaser, or a for-one pleaser. It pleases, OK? I've subbed the classic use of anchovies with my favorite plant-based fish-y food, dulse, and it's a dead ringer. Add some briney olives and capers and a boatload of parsley and you'll see why it's the ultimate palate pleaser.

SERVES 2 GENEROUSLY

INGREDIENTS

1 box of gluten-free spaghetti or capellini

2 tablespoons olive oil

4 cloves garlic, roughly chopped

1 jar of your favorite marinara sauce

¼ cup dulse leaves chopped or dulse flakes

1 cup kalamata or black olives, pitted and roughly chopped

½ teaspoon red chili flakes, optional

Sea salt and pepper to taste

1 cup chopped fresh parsley

3 tablespoons capers

Good olive oil for drizzling

METHOD

Cook the pasta as directed. Drain and let cool. If using gluten-free pasta, rinse under cold water immediately to prevent gumminess.

In a large shallow pan, add the oil and garlic. Sauté for 3 minutes on medium heat, then add the marinara sauce. Bring to a boil, then lower to simmer. Add the dulse, olives, and chili flakes. Cover and simmer for 10 minutes. Taste the sauce and season with salt and pepper as needed. Add the cooked pasta and toss it in the sauce. Add the parsley and capers and toss. Serve hot, drizzled with olive oil.

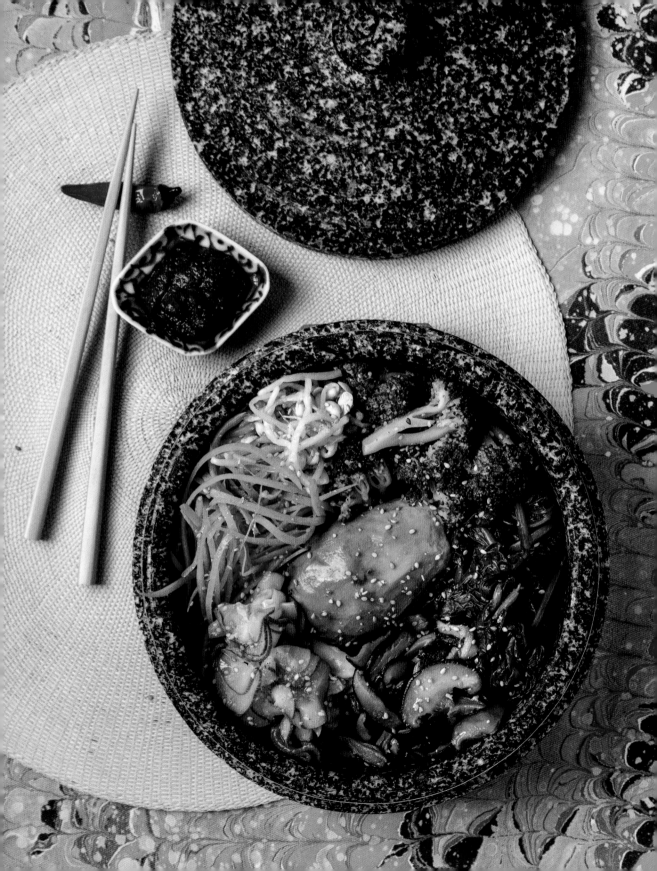

QUINOA BIBIMBAP

This is the dish of my childhood, though my mother never really made it for me at home. In northern New Jersey, Korean Americans abound, so we ate out at Korean restaurants a lot. Yes, there would be galbi (marinated short rib) and bulgogi (salty-sweet beef) on the grill, and an *ajumma* gruffly wielding kitchen scissors to cut up the meat and slap it onto our plates. While my brothers reveled in their carnivorous glory, however, my favorite thing to order was this naturally vegetarian dish. A little more refined and truly like a little personal party at your plate, brought to you in a sizzling *dolsot*, or agalmatolite pot, so hot that if you touched it, you'd burn your fingers—like, actually burn them. (The trade-off is the scorched crispy rice you earn, with a little elbow grease, at the bottom of the pot.) You can certainly use rice here as the base—ideally, short grain white or brown rice. But I think quinoa lightens the dish up a bit. If you're going to be entertaining, a dolsot makes quite a statement. You can invest in one of your own and, with a brush of sesame oil over an open flame for about 10 minutes, create that elusive crispy bottom. (A cast-iron pan will work here too.) If there are leftovers, do as my mom did and sauté everything in a frying pan the next day with kimchi or gochujang and make a really spicy fried rice served with lettuce leaves to wrap.

SERVES 2 TO 4

INGREDIENTS

2 cups (60 g) packed baby spinach

2 cups (140 g) broccoli florets

2 large carrots (140 g), cut into matchsticks or shredded with a julienne peeler

2 cups (370 g) bean sprouts

2 small zucchini (236 g), thinly sliced into half-moons

1 tablespoon avocado oil

2 cups (200 g) shiitake mushrooms caps

1 tablespoon tamari sauce

1 teaspoon toasted sesame oil

½ teaspoon toasted sesame oil

½ teaspoon sesame seeds or gomasio

Dash of sea salt

2½ cups (425 g) cooked white quinoa

Garnish

Sliced avocado

¼ cup (58 g/1.71 ounces) vegan kimchi

½ cup (120 ml) Beet Gochujang (page 235)

METHOD

Fill a deep pan or medium pot with 1 inch (2.5 cm) water. Place a steamer basket inside and bring the water to a boil. One vegetable at a time, add the spinach, broccoli, carrots, sprouts, and zucchini to the basket and blanch for about 3 minutes, until cooked but still al dente. Set each vegetable aside in a separate bowl to cool.

In a separate pan, heat the avocado oil. Add the shiitakes, tamari, and 1 teaspoon of the sesame oil and sauté until browned, 3 to 5 minutes. Set aside to cool.

Once the steamed vegetables are cool, drizzle ½ teaspoon of the remaining sesame oil, ½ teaspoon of the sesame seeds, and a dash of salt into each bowl. Gently massage the veggies with your hands so that the seasoning is evenly distributed.

For plating, scoop ½ cup to 1 cup (92 g to 185 g) cooked quinoa into individual-size serving bowls or stone bowls and arrange ¼ cup or a small handful of each vegetable (broccoli, spinach, carrots, bean sprouts, zucchini and sautéed shiitakes) around the perimeter. Add the avocado, kimchi, and a dollop of gochujang, and serve!

CRISPY ONE-PAN KALE KIMCHI RICE

his dish will always say "home" for me. One of my mom's favorite things to make for herself was and still is kimchi fried rice. Usually using the dregs of our leftovers, she'd dump a whole load of spicy kimchi with day-old rice into the pan and fry it up to perfection. This recipe takes it an extra step by crisping up the bottom—an homage to those sizzling bibimbaps, but less work and in one pan, so whoever is doing the dishes won't be so mad that you'll have ruined only one pan. Sometimes I like to put this rice in a nori wrap with a ton of raw greens for a quick, satisfying dinner.

SERVES 4

INGREDIENTS

2 tablespoons avocado oil

4 cloves garlic, minced

½ white onion (170 g), minced

2 teaspoons grated ginger

2 cups (180 g) shiitake mushrooms, thinly sliced

1 cup (100 g) bean sprouts

3 teaspoons toasted sesame oil

2 tablespoons tamari

1 bunch lacinato kale (274 g), destemmed and thinly sliced

2 large carrots (133 g), peeled and shredded

1 (16-ounce/453-g) jar kimchi, or 2 cups (300 g) chopped

1 cup (185 g) brown rice, or 2 cups cooked (13½ ounces/385 g)

3 scallions, thinly sliced

Sea salt and black pepper (optional)

Garnish

Sesame seeds

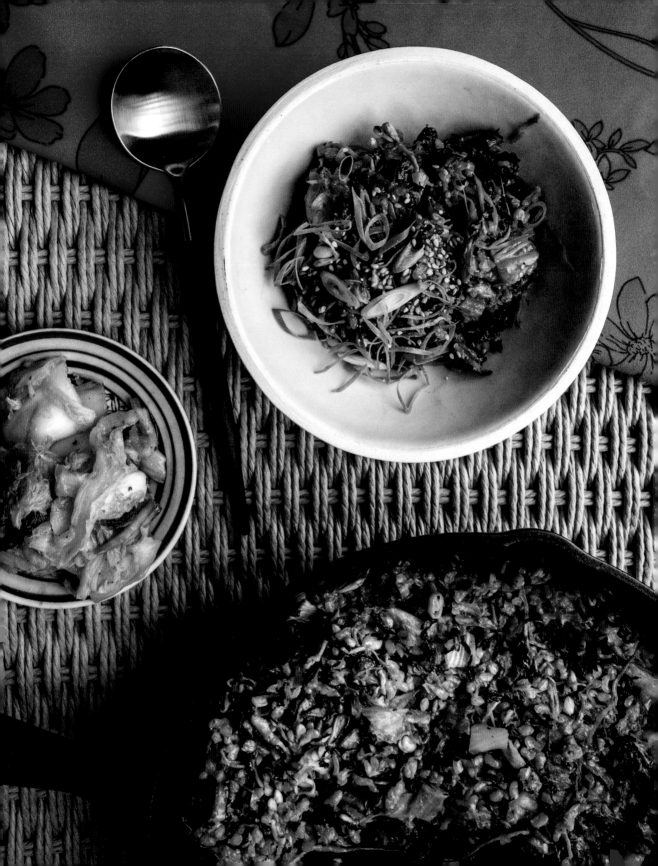

METHOD

In a cast-iron pan, heat the oil. Add the garlic, onion, ginger, mushrooms, sprouts, 1 teaspoon of the toasted sesame oil, and tamari and sauté on medium-low heat until browned, about 5 to 7 minutes. Add the kale and carrots and cook until it wilts, about 1 minute.

Add the kimchi and the remaining juice in the jar. Increase the heat and sauté for 2 to 3 minutes, until the flavors combine. Add the cooked rice and scallions and stir well, so that the veggies and kimchi are evenly distributed. Season with salt and pepper, if needed. Keep on the heat for 3 minutes more, stirring occasionally to prevent sticking.

Transfer the rice to a bowl. You can stop here! But if you want a crispy bottom, brush the remaining 2 teaspoons of sesame oil onto the bottom of the pan. Transfer the rice back to the pan, spreading it out evenly. Let sit on low heat, uncovered, for about 3 minutes. Resist the urge to check, but you want to hear a soft sizzle. Remove from the heat and let sit for 3 to 5 minutes. Garnish with sesame seeds and scallions. Serve.

Note: For less mushy fried rice, make the rice a day before and refrigerate.

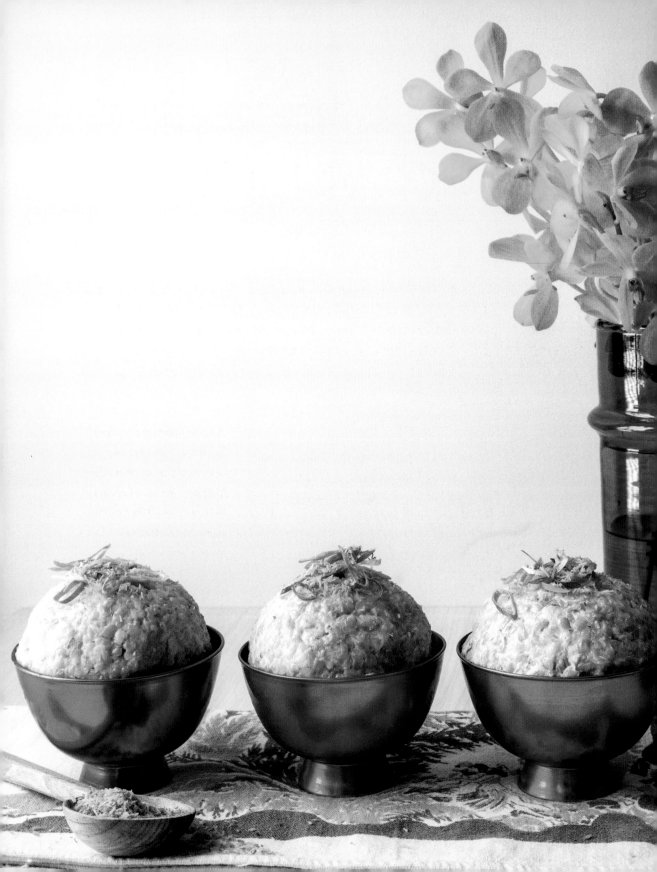

CREAMY COCONUT BROWN RICE

This is an homage to my favorite rice dish at a now-shuttered New York City institution, Sushi Samba. Very *Sex and the City*, very early aughts, this was a see-and-be-seen type of place that secretly had the most luscious, creamy, salty-and-slightly-sweet coconut rice there ever was. My mouth waters when I just think about it. I typically would order it with some crunchy, garlicky sautéed collard greens and black beans, and I would and still do call that the perfect meal.

SERVES 4

INGREDIENTS

1½ cups (11 ounces/310 g) brown rice (long or short grain)

1 tablespoon coconut oil

1 teaspoon sea salt, plus more if needed

1 (13½-ounce/398-ml) can unsweetened coconut milk

1 teaspoon coconut sugar

3 scallions, chopped

¼ cup (19 g) shredded unsweetened coconut

Freshly cracked black pepper (optional)

METHOD

Soak the rice for 2 hours or overnight in 2 cups (480 ml) water at room temperature. When ready, drain. In a large pot, heat the coconut oil. Add the rice and toast on medium-low heat for about 3 minutes, being careful not to burn the rice, but enough so you smell a fragrant, nutty aroma. Add 3½ cups (840 ml) water and the salt, bring to a boil, and then simmer, covered, for 30 minutes, or until the liquid has been absorbed and the rice is tender.

Add the milk to the pot and bring to a boil, then simmer, uncovered, on medium-low heat for 5 minutes. Continue to stir to prevent the rice from sticking to the bottom. If you feel the rice is dry, add ¼ cup water and stir. Add the sugar, half the scallions, and half the shredded coconut and stir. In a dry pan, quickly toast the remaining coconut until lightly browned and fragrant, about 2 minutes. Transfer the coconut rice to a serving bowl and top with the remaining scallions and the toasted coconut. Season with salt and pepper, if needed.

SPINACH DILL RICE

By far my favorite rice dish. Hearty, herby, slightly crunchy and tart, it hits all the right spots. Maybe because you can sneak in a boatload of greens without anyone really being the wiser.

SERVES 2 TO 4

INGREDIENTS

1 cup (195 g) dried white long-grain rice (I like basmati for this.)

Sea salt

2 tablespoons olive oil

1 clove garlic, grated

½ large chopped yellow or white onion, or 1 cup chopped (75 g)

4 cups (120 g) roughly chopped spinach

Freshly cracked black pepper

1 cup (9 g) chopped fresh dill

4 scallions, chopped

Juice of 1 lemon, or 2 tablespoons lemon juice

METHOD

Rinse the rice in cool water until the water runs clear. Drain the rice, then place it in a medium pot. Add 1¾ cups (420 ml) water and ½ teaspoon salt. Bring to a boil and simmer, covered, for 10 minutes, stirring occasionally to prevent the rice from sticking to the bottom.

Remove the pot from the heat and leave covered for 10 minutes more. Transfer the rice to a bowl. In the same pot, combine the oil, garlic, and onion and sauté on medium-low heat until fragrant, 3 to 4 minutes. Add the spinach and continue to stir until it cooks down, 3 minutes more. Season with salt and pepper to taste. Add the cooked rice and stir until well mixed. Add the dill, scallions, and lemon juice and stir until blended. Turn off the heat and season with more salt and pepper, if needed.

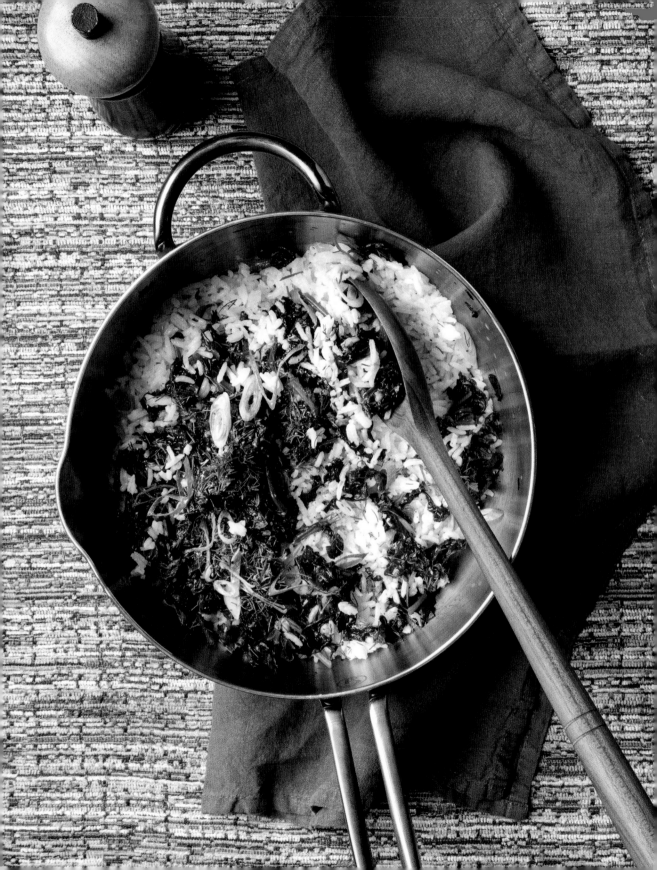

RIGATONI ALLA VODKA

Growing up in New Jersey, I had plenty of Italian American joints to choose from, and each one had its version of penne alla vodka. I learned about the dish in high school and you would find it on every menu—in some places, even as a pizza topping. Believe it or not, this version is as creamy and decadent as the original, sans the cream and the vodka (which, curiously, I don't really think was in there to begin with).

SERVES 4

INGREDIENTS

For the pasta

1 (12-ounce/340-g) package gluten-free rigatoni or penne

1 teaspoon sea salt

For the sauce

2 tablespoons olive oil

3 cloves garlic, minced

2 cups (480 ml) your favorite store-bought marinara sauce

1 cup (240 ml) unsweetened, unflavored plant-based milk

½ teaspoon chili flakes

½ cup (30 g) nutritional yeast

1 clove garlic, grated

Sea salt

Freshly cracked black pepper

METHOD

Make the pasta: Fill a large pot with 6 to 7 cups (1.4 L to 1.7 L) water, add the salt, and bring to a boil. Add the rigatoni. Boil for 12 to 14 minutes, until tender but still slightly al dente. Drain and immediately rinse with cold water. Set aside.

Make the sauce: In a large pot, heat the oil. Add the minced garlic and sauté on medium-high heat until fragrant, about 3 minutes. Add the marinara, milk, chili flakes, and yeast and bring to a boil. Simmer for 5 minutes. Add the grated garlic and season with salt and pepper to taste. Add the rigatoni and stir. Let simmer on low for 5 minutes more. Serve hot.

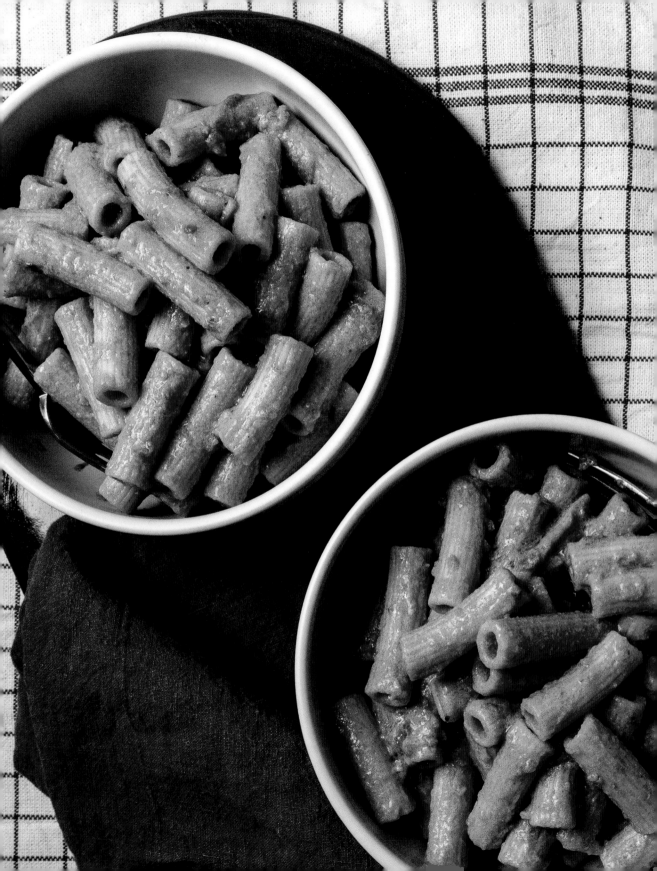

PENNE WITH SHIITAKE CRUMBLES AND BROCCOLI RABE

This is the kind of dish you can serve to a devoted meat eater and not get any complaints. I infuse the shiitakes with all the aromatics you find in a classic sausage via the peppery bitterness of the broccoli rabe, arguably my favorite vegetable. You could add a red sauce here, but I think the flavors stand wonderfully on their own.

SERVES 2 TO 4

INGREDIENTS

3 teaspoons sea salt

1 (12-ounce/340-g) package gluten-free penne

1 bunch broccoli rabe, stems trimmed

3 tablespoons olive oil

4 cloves garlic, thinly sliced

Juice and zest of 1 lemon

For the shiitake crumbles

2 tablespoons avocado oil

3 cloves garlic, minced

½ teaspoon ground cumin

1 teaspoon fennel seeds

2 cups (194 g) shiitake mushrooms, destemmed and caps roughly chopped

1 tablespoon tamari

½ teaspoon red chili flakes

Sea salt and freshly cracked black pepper (optional)

METHOD

Fill a large pot with 6 to 7 cups (1.4 L to 1.7 L) water, add 1 teaspoon of the salt, and bring to a boil. Add the penne and boil for 13 to 15 minutes, until cooked but slightly al dente. Drain and immediately rinse with cold water. Set aside.

Fill a separate pot with 4 to 5 cups (960 ml to 1.2 L) water, add the remaining 2 teaspoons salt, and bring to a boil. Add the broccoli rabe, submerging it in the water, and simmer, uncovered, for 10 minutes. Drain and let cool, then roughly chop. Set aside.

Make the shiitake crumbles: In a shallow pan, heat the avocado oil on medium high. Add the garlic, cumin, and fennel seeds and sauté for about 2 minutes. Add the mushrooms, tamari, and chili flakes and sauté on medium heat for 4 to 5 minutes, until browned. Add water if needed, and use a wooden spoon to stir, to prevent sticking at the bottom. Season with salt and pepper, if needed. Set aside.

In a large pan, heat the olive oil on medium high. Add the sliced garlic and sauté for 1 to 2 minutes, until fragrant but not browned. Add the broccoli rabe, shiitake crumbles, and penne and stir on medium heat to combine well. Add the lemon juice and zest and season with more salt and pepper, if needed. Transfer to a serving platter, and serve hot.

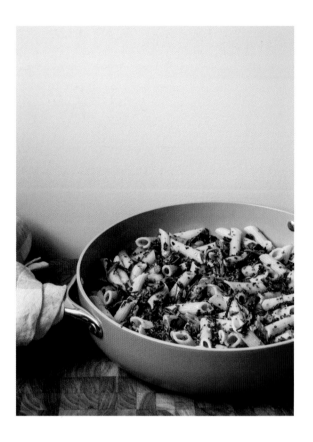

GREEN PESTO LASAGNA

There is arguably nothing more comforting than lasagna. I remember going out with my childhood babysitter Sally to an Italian joint in New Jersey called Spaghett-ta-ta. Can't make those names up, can you? I always ordered the lasagna. It came in a scalding-hot personal casserole dish, and the best part by far was the bubbly insides and the crispy edges. I can still taste them! This is my green-ified homage, and it's just as decadent and comforting.

SERVES 4 TO 6

INGREDIENTS

1 (9-ounce/255-g) package gluten-free lasagna noodles

Olive oil, for rubbing on the noodles

3 to 4 zucchini, thinly sliced lengthwise

1 cup (246 g) Cashew Ricotta (page 228)

2 cups (225 g) chopped spinach or kale

Toppings

Olive oil

Fresh basil leaves

Flaky sea salt

Freshly cracked black pepper

For the pesto

2 cups (225 g) chopped spinach or kale

2 cups (225 g) arugula

4 to 5 cloves garlic

1 cup (24 g) fresh basil

Juice and zest of 1 lemon

¼ cup (15 g) nutritional yeast

½ cup (120 ml) olive oil

½ teaspoon sea salt

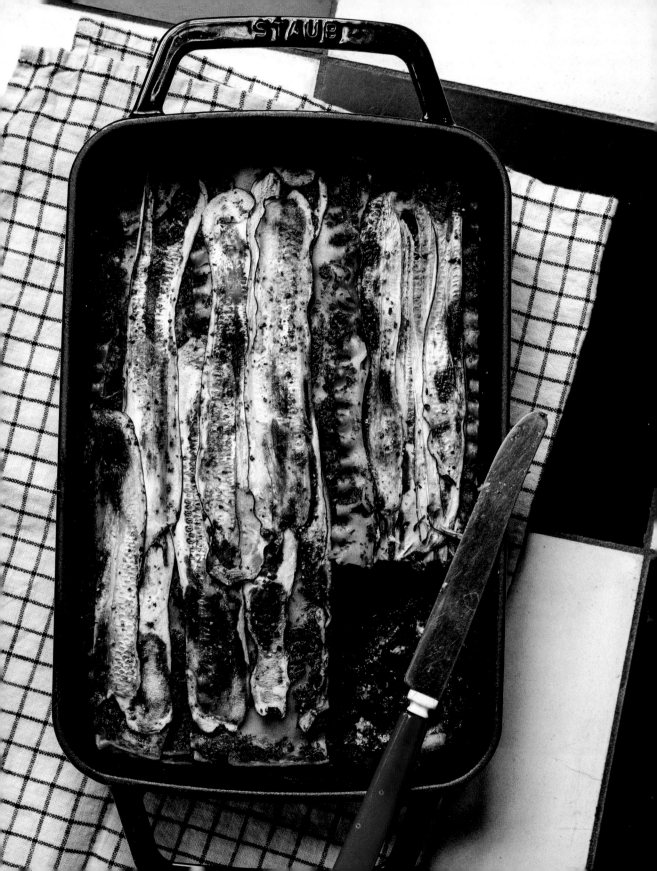

METHOD

Preheat the oven to 375°F (190°C). Fill a large pot with 5 to 6 cups (1.2 L to 1.4 L) salted water and bring to a boil. Add the noodles and boil for 4 to 5 minutes. Drain and rub with a little olive oil and lay out on a dish towel over a flat surface.

Make the pesto: In a food processor, blend all the pesto ingredients until creamy.

In a casserole dish or lasagna pan, spoon ½ cup of pesto onto the bottom and spread evenly. Add one layer of noodles, then another spoon of pesto, followed by one layer of the zucchini, then one spoon of cashew ricotta spread evenly over the zucchini. Sprinkle a layer of the spinach, then add a layer of noodles and repeat. Finish with a layer of zucchini. Brush olive oil on top and sprinkle with the basil and salt and pepper to taste. Cover the dish tightly with a lid or tin foil and bake for 45 to 50 minutes. Uncover for the last 10 minutes, to brown. Let sit for 10 minutes before serving.

PORTOBELLO AND EGGPLANT BANH MI

 s far as sandwiches go, the banh mi is hard to beat. The crusty bread, slathered in garlicky aioli with abundant veggies and bright herbs punctuated with pickled goodness. Can you get better than that? I think not.

MAKES 2 LARGE SANDWICHES

INGREDIENTS

For the pickled vegetables

¾ cup (180 ml) apple cider vinegar

1 teaspoon coconut sugar

½ teaspoon sea salt

1 clove garlic, grated

½ cup (148 g) thinly sliced daikon radish

2 carrots, peeled and cut into matchsticks

2 Persian cucumbers, thinly sliced (½ cup/60 g)

1 cup (90 g) napa cabbage

For the eggplant and mushroom

1 medium eggplant (550 g)

1 teaspoon sea salt (for eggplant)

2 tablespoons avocado oil

2 teaspoons toasted sesame oil

2 teaspoons tamari

2 portobello mushroom caps

For the aioli

½ cup (120 ml) Aquafaba Mayo (page 223)

½ jalapeño chile, seeded and chopped

Zest of 1 lime

Juice of ½ lime

1 clove garlic, grated

½ teaspoon sea salt

Freshly cracked black pepper

For assembling

1 baguette or 2 gluten-free rolls, cut in half

1 clove garlic, halved

½ cup (39 g) packed fresh cilantro

½ cup (28 g) fresh basil

½ cup (14 g) fresh mint

¼ cup (55 g) Chopped Liver (page 236; optional)

1 lime, quartered

METHOD

Preheat the oven to 400°F (205°C).

Make the pickled vegetables: In a medium bowl, whisk together the vinegar, sugar, salt, and garlic and ½ cup (120 ml) water. Arrange the daikon, carrots, cucumber, and cabbage in separate small bowls and pour the pickling solution evenly into each bowl. Let sit for 20 to 30 minutes.

Prepare the eggplant and mushrooms: Using a vegetable peeler, peel the eggplant lengthwise every other inch (2.5 cm) or so to form zebra-like stripes. Then slice it into ½-inch (12-mm) rounds. Arrange the rounds on a dish towel on a flat surface and sprinkle the salt evenly over them. Let sit for 15 minutes to sweat. Pat dry with a dish towel. Drizzle the rounds with the avocado oil, 1 teaspoon of the sesame oil, and 1 teaspoon of the tamari.

In a shallow bowl, massage the portobello caps with the remaining 1 teaspoon of the sesame oil and the remaining 1 teaspoon of the tamari. On a parchment-lined baking sheet, arrange the cap face up with the eggplant rounds. Roast for 10 minutes, flip the cap and rounds, and roast for 10 minutes more. Let cool and slice in half.

Make the aioli: In a small bowl, combine the mayo, jalapeño, lime zest and juice, garlic, and salt and whisk together. Season with pepper to taste. Transfer to a small serving bowl or ramekin.

Assemble the sandwiches: Lightly toast the halves of the baguette. Rub each half of the bread with a halved garlic clove. Spread 1 tablespoon of the aioli on each half. Add sliced portobello cap, eggplant rounds, pickled veggies, and the cilantro, basil, mint, and a schmear of chopped liver, if using. Serve with lime wedges.

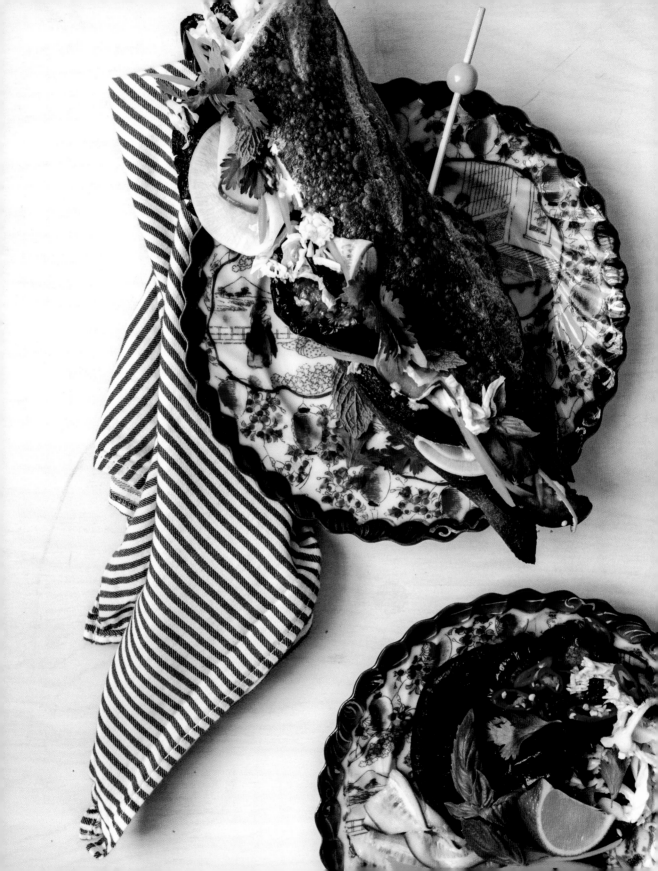

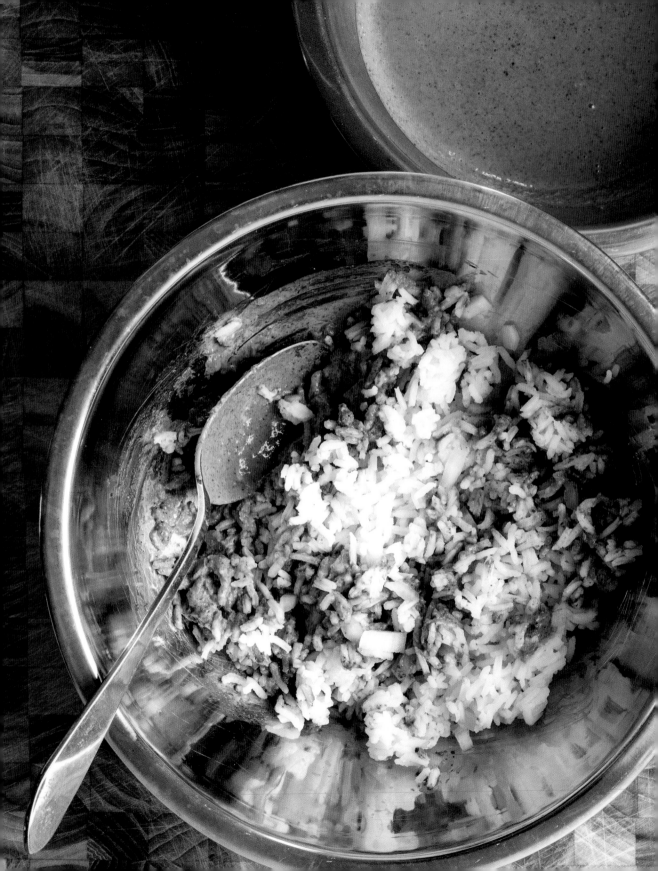

CREAMY CILANTRO RICE

T his rice dish is in regular rotation in our home. It's the perfect side for taco night or with a crunchy, hydrating salad. You could also serve it with stewed black beans for a grounding, hearty plant-based meal. I love the versatility of this dish and have been known to swap in other herbs like parsley, mint, or dill to change it up.

SERVES 4

INGREDIENTS

2 cups (360 g) basmati rice (jasmine or brown will work well here too)

4 cups (360 g) filtered water

½ teaspoon salt

½ red onion, minced

Cilantro Sauce:

1 entire bunch organic cilantro, rinsed and patted dry

2 cloves garlic

Juice of 1 lime

½ jalapeño (keep the seeds if you like it spicy)

¼ cup olive oil or avocado oil

Salt and pepper to taste

METHOD

Rinse the rice in a colander under cold water until the water runs clear. Drain. In a large pot, add the rinsed rice, water, and salt. Bring to a boil, then simmer, covered, until the rice is cooked, mixing occasionally, about 20 minutes (35 to 40 minutes if using brown rice). Remove from the heat and fluff immediately; set aside.

While the rice is cooking, combine the cilantro, garlic, lime juice, jalapeño, and oil in a food processor or blender. Blend, slowly adding in water until you achieve a creamy, liquid consistency. Season with salt and pepper as needed. Pour the sauce into the pot with the cooked rice and mix well until the rice is fully coated, until you achieve a creamy risotto-like consistency. Serve warm.

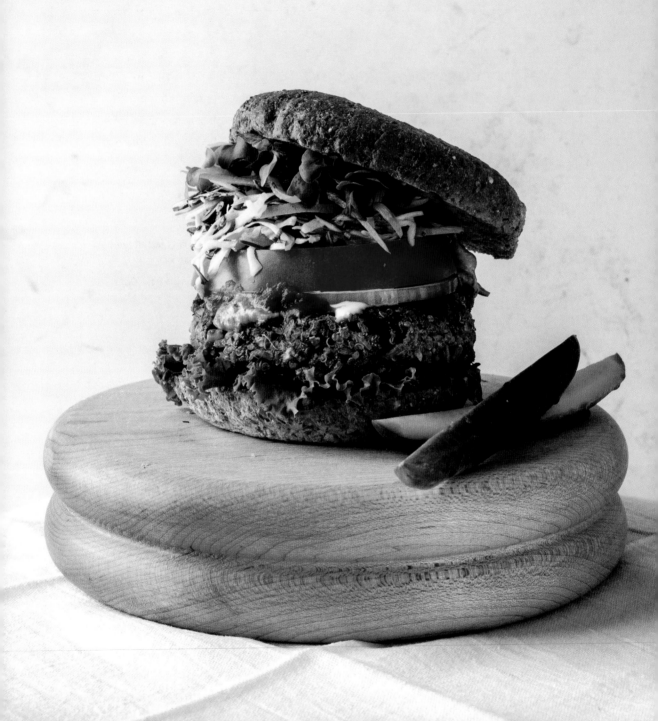

JUICE PULP BURGERS

'm often asked what to do with the leftover pulp of daily veggie juice. There are plenty of ways to repurpose, rather than discard, the fibrous, rainbow-colored pulp from a vibrant juice blend. Enter homemade veggie burgers! These nutrient-packed patties get crispy on the outside and remain moist and chewy on the inside—exactly how I like 'em. Reducing food waste makes these all the more worthwhile.

MAKES 10 TO 12 BURGERS, DEPENDING ON DESIRED THICKNESS

INGREDIENTS

For the burgers

1 tablespoon ground flax seeds

2½ tablespoons warm water

2 cups (205 g) juice pulp (from any juice without fruit: beets, carrots, kale, parsley, celery, fennel)

½ cup (205 g) cooked brown rice

½ cup (85 g) cooked quinoa

½ cup (95 g) white rice flour

½ cup (85 g) canned water chestnuts, drained and chopped

½ sweet onion, minced (5 ounces/135 g)

¼ cup (90 g) frozen sweet peas, thawed

2 tablespoons chopped fresh dill

¼ cup (30 g) frozen corn kernels, thawed (optional)

Sea salt

Black pepper

Fixings

Food for Life Ezekiel 4:9 Sprouted Grain Burger Buns

Aquafaba mayo (page 223)

Organic ketchup

Grainy mustard

Sprouts or microgreens

Sauerkraut

Tomato, lettuce, onion

Pickle

METHOD

Preheat the oven to 400°F (205°C). Combine the flax seeds and warm water. Wait until it forms the consistency of an egg. Meanwhile, in a large bowl, combine juice pulp, rice, quinoa, rice flour, water chestnuts, onion, peas, dill, and flax egg and massage well with your hands until the mixture has a burger meat–like consistency. Mix in the corn if using. Season with salt and pepper. Scoop ¼ cup (37.25 g) (or ½ cup/75 g for larger burgers) of the burger mixture, form patties with your hands, and transfer to a parchment-lined baking sheet. Bake for 15 minutes, flip, and bake for another 20 minutes, until browned.

Serve buns with mayo, ketchup, mustard, sprouts, kraut, tomato, lettuce, and onion with a side pickle.

MAITAKE AND BRUSSELS TACOS

love tacos. So much. It's actually a miracle there is only one taco recipe in this book because I'd happily include a chapter full of tacos. This one just happens to be my favorite, mostly because the combo really hits the spot. I even included this dish on the menu at a pop-up I did at Las Ventanas al Paraíso, a Rosewood Resort in Cabo San Lucas, and if a taco dish stands the test of time in Mexico, well then, I think it's a go.

SERVES 2 TO 4

INGREDIENTS

1 cup (90 g) shredded or thinly sliced red cabbage

2 cups (230 g) trimmed and halved brussels sprouts

2 cups (165 g) shiitake mushrooms, stems removed

2 cups (155 g) trumpet mushrooms, ends trimmed, sliced lengthwise into thirds

2 cups (175 g) maitake mushrooms, ends trimmed

3 tablespoons avocado oil

½ teaspoon ground cumin

½ teaspoon sea salt

Freshly cracked black pepper

1 (8-ounce/227-g) can water chestnuts

6 to 8 sprouted corn or grain-free tortillas

For the pickled cabbage

¼ cup (60 ml) apple cider vinegar

½ cup (120 ml) filtered water

2 teaspoons coconut sugar

2 teaspoons sea salt

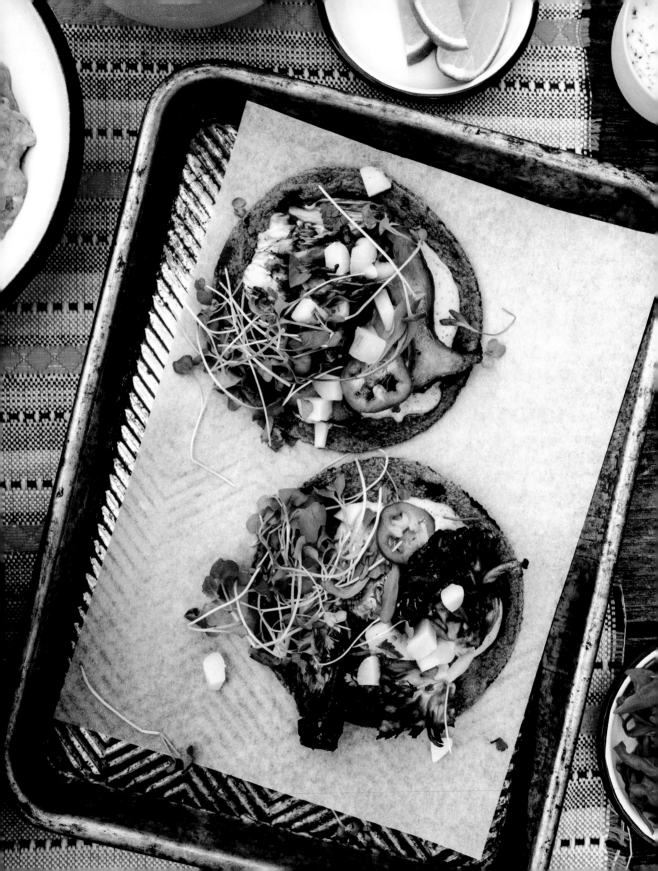

ASSEMBLY

6 to 8 tablespoons Cilantro Jalapeño Aioli (recipe below)

Microgreens

Lime wedge

METHOD

Preheat the oven to 400°F (205°C).

Make the pickled cabbage: Whisk together the vinegar, water, sugar, and sea salt in a medium bowl. Add the cabbage and let sit for 20 minutes to an hour. (You can also prepare this the night before!)

To both the brussels and the mushrooms, add 1 ½ tablespoons avocado oil, ½ teaspoon ground cumin, and salt and pepper to taste. Massage well with your hands. Roast on a parchment-lined baking sheet for 15 minutes, until browned. Let cool.

While the vegetables are cooking, drain and roughly chop the water chestnuts. Drain the pickled cabbage and place in a small bowl.

Place the tortillas on a low flame over the stovetop (if you don't have a gas stove, place on a pan to warm, 2 minutes on each side) and let char on each side for 5 to 10 seconds.

To assemble the tacos: Schmear 1 tablespoon aioli onto a tortilla. Add a handful of brussels and mushrooms, sprinkle with water chestnuts, top with red cabbage slaw and microgreens, and serve with a lime wedge. Enjoy immediately.

CILANTRO JALAPEÑO AIOLI

MAKES 1 CUP

INGREDIENTS

1 cup (240 ml) Aquafaba Mayo (page 223)

1 clove garlic, grated

Juice of 1 lime

½ jalapeño chile, seeded and chopped

1 bunch cilantro, roughly chopped

Sea salt

Optional

½ teaspoon chili powder

In a small bowl, add mayo, garlic, lime juice, jalapeño, cilantro, and chili powder (if using). Mix well. Season with salt.

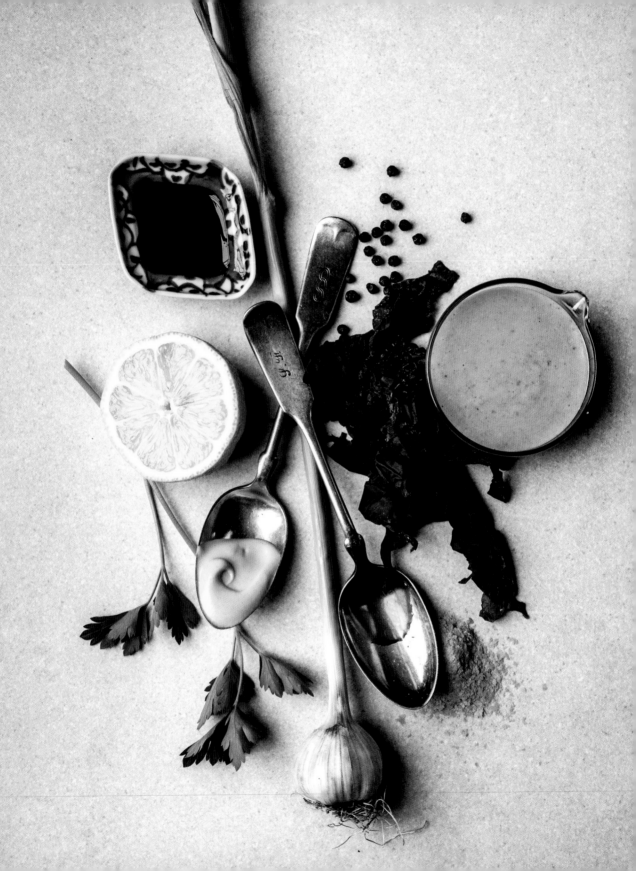

DRESSINGS, DIPS, AND SPREADS

BISTRO SHALLOT VINAIGRETTE

I once read that food writer David Lebovitz's secret for a perfect French vinaigrette is to pickle the shallots. All you need to do is let them sit in vinegar (here, apple cider vinegar) to lend the dressing a nuance that you wouldn't be able to identify if I hadn't just told you. I haven't made dressings differently since. There's no going back.

MAKES 1¼ CUPS (300 ML) DRESSING

INGREDIENTS

1 shallot (2½ ounces/70 g), peeled and minced

¼ cup (60 ml) apple cider vinegar

2 tablespoons chopped fresh parsley

2 tablespoons chopped fresh tarragon

2 tablespoons Dijon mustard

¾ cup (180 ml) olive oil

2 tablespoons capers

1 teaspoon sea salt

Freshly cracked black pepper

METHOD

In a medium mixing bowl, combine the shallot and vinegar and let sit to pickle for at least 15 minutes or up to an hour. Add the parsley, tarragon, mustard, oil, capers, salt, and ¼ cup (60 ml) water to the bowl and whisk well. Season with pepper to taste. Use the dressing immediately or save it in an airtight container in the fridge for 5 days. Note: Oil will harden in the fridge, so bring to room temperature before using.

BASIC VINAIGRETTE

This is the dressing to have in your fridge for those quickie salad moments. You can perk it up with any herb or other additions, but, really, the simpler the better.

MAKES 1 CUP (240 ML) DRESSING

INGREDIENTS

½ cup (120 ml) olive oil

2 tablespoons apple cider vinegar

½ cup (120 ml) filtered water

1 tablespoon Dijon mustard

1 clove garlic, grated

½ teaspoon sea salt

2 tablespoons fresh lemon juice

METHOD

In a bowl, whisk all the ingredients. Store the dressing in the fridge in an airtight container for up to a week.

Optional: For a slightly sweeter vinaigrette, can add 1 tablespoon of raw honey or maple syrup.

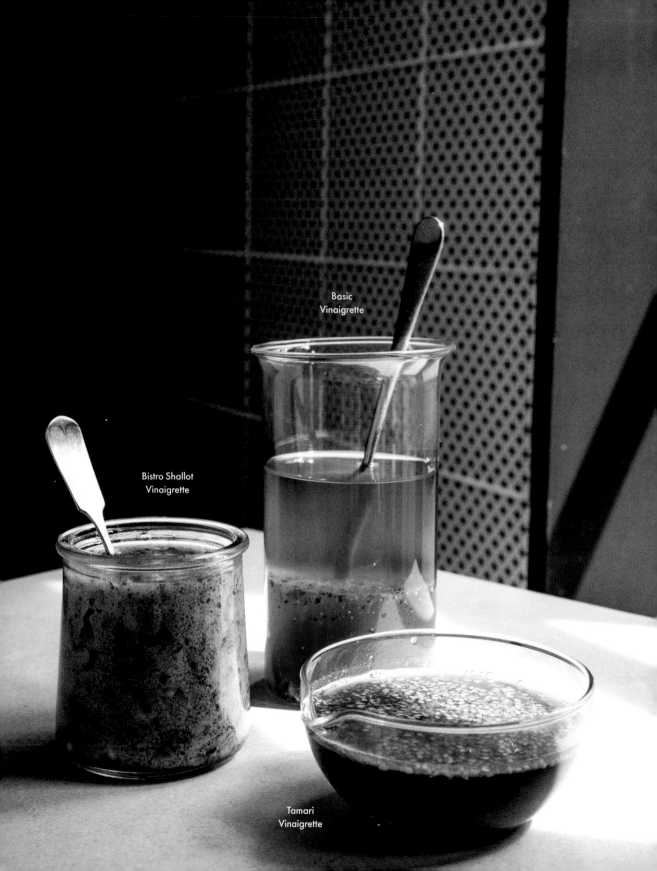

Basic
Vinaigrette

Bistro Shallot
Vinaigrette

Tamari
Vinaigrette

TAMARI VINAIGRETTE

I probably use this dressing at least once a day. It's simple, easy, and to the point, and truly goes with everything. The tamari and toasted sesame oil add a little Asian flair, but I use the dressing on any salad, with any meal—it's that versatile.

MAKES 1½ CUPS (360 ML) DRESSING

INGREDIENTS

¼ cup (60 ml) rice vinegar or apple cider vinegar

2 teaspoons toasted sesame oil

½ cup (120 ml) Vegan Dashi Broth (page 157) or water

3 to 4 tablespoons tamari

1 tablespoon maple syrup

1 teaspoon sesame seeds

METHOD

In a bowl, whisk all the ingredients with ¼ cup (60 ml) water, if using dashi. (If using water in place of dashi, omit.) Store the dressing in an airtight container in the fridge for up to a week.

DULSE CAESAR

The Caesar is the king of all salads. Done well, it never disappoints. Done half well, it doesn't disappoint. There are countless versions and riffs on it, particularly in the plant-based world, but this dressing, which incorporates umami-rich dulse and tamari, really recalls the classic one we all grew up with.

MAKES 1¼ CUPS (300 ML) DRESSING

INGREDIENTS

4 large cloves garlic

¼ cup (½ ounce/14 g) packed dulse leaves, or 2 large sheets toasted nori

2 tablespoons nutritional yeast

¼ cup (2½ ounces/70 g) fresh parsley leaves

2 tablespoons tamari or coconut aminos

Juice of 3 lemons, or ¼ cup (60 ml) lemon juice

1 tablespoon Dijon mustard

½ teaspoon sea salt, or more to taste

¼ teaspoon ground black pepper

½ cup (120 ml) olive oil

¼ cup (60 ml) cold filtered water

Freshly cracked black pepper

METHOD

In a food processor or blender, blend the garlic, dulse, yeast, parsley, tamari, lemon juice, mustard, salt, pepper, olive oil, and water until creamy. Season with more salt and pepper to taste. The dressing is best if it's super peppery, in my humble opinion. It will keep in the fridge in an airtight container for up to 5 days.

If you cannot find dulse seaweed, you can substitute toasted nori, which is a good dupe. But it won't capture the same pungent "anchovy" flavor.

THE UNIVERSAL

The name says it all. This dressing goes with everything: salads, steamed veggies, rice, toast—literally everything! It's an homage to that yogi-like dressing you find at hippie joints and plant-based cafés around the globe, the one where you can't put your finger on what's in it, but you could literally drink it. Granola in the best way. Sound familiar? Now make it stat.

MAKES 1 CUP (240 ML) DRESSING

INGREDIENTS

¼ cup tahini

⅓ cup (75 ml) ice water

½ cup (120 ml) olive oil

1 bunch dill

1 bunch chives

2 cloves garlic

Juice of 1 lemon, or
2 tablespoons lemon juice

2 tablespoons tamari

2 tablespoons apple
cider vinegar

½ teaspoon sea salt

Freshly cracked black pepper

METHOD

In a food processor, blend the tahini, ice water, oil, dill, chives, garlic, lemon juice, tamari, vinegar, and salt until creamy. Season with pepper to taste. The dressing will keep in the fridge in an airtight container for up to 3 days.

ITALIAN HOUSE DRESSING

You know the restaurants where they ask your dressing preference—"Thousand Island, Ranch, or Italian House"? This is the last one. The elusive tangy, herby dressing that goes well on any salad or sandwich, and that is great to keep in the fridge to put on anything, really.

MAKES 1 CUP (240 ML) DRESSING

INGREDIENTS

½ cup (120 ml) olive oil

2 tablespoons apple
cider vinegar

1 tablespoon dried oregano

1 clove garlic, grated

½ teaspoon sea salt

2 tablespoons chopped
fresh parsley

¼ cup (60 ml) filtered water

METHOD

In a bowl, whisk all the ingredients. Store the dressing in the fridge in an airtight container for up to a week.

JAPANESE HOUSE

The classic dressing you get at most casual Japanese joints, bright thanks to the ginger, slightly sweet from the carrots and satisfyingly grainy—perfect to cling to sturdy lettuces, especially the classic Japanese House Salad (page 85).

MAKES 2 CUPS (480 ML) DRESSING

INGREDIENTS

4 large carrots

3-inch (7.5-cm) knob ginger (½ ounce/14 g), peeled

½ large sweet onion (4½ ounces/130 g)

2 tablespoons unsweetened creamy peanut butter

¾ cup (180 ml) avocado oil

2 tablespoons tamari

3 tablespoons rice vinegar

1 tablespoon maple syrup

2 teaspoons toasted sesame oil

½ teaspoon sea salt

1 tablespoon white miso

1 clove garlic

METHOD

In a blender or food processor, blend all the ingredients with ¼ cup (60 ml) water, or more if needed, until creamy. You can keep the dressing in the fridge in an airtight container for up to 1 week.

LIQUID GOLD

This dressing is just as the name describes—liquid gold. It's easy to keep in the fridge for the week to put on salads or serve as a dip, and it's pretty universal. It reminds me of the dressing you get at any Middle Eastern restaurant—perfectly light, slightly creamy, and spiced in a way that you can't put your finger on but that makes the vegetables taste even more delicious.

MAKES 1 CUP (240 ML) DRESSING

INGREDIENTS

¼ cup (60 ml) tahini

¾ cup (180 ml) ice water

2 ice cubes

¼ cup (60 ml) olive oil

1 clove garlic, grated

½ teaspoon berbere seasoning, smoked paprika, or sumac

½ teaspoon ground turmeric

2 tablespoons lemon juice

1 teaspoon sea salt

Freshly cracked black pepper

METHOD

In a medium bowl, whisk the tahini, ice water, ice cubes, oil, garlic, berbere seasoning, turmeric, lemon juice, and salt. Season with pepper to taste. Transfer the dressing to an airtight container and keep in the fridge for up to 3 days.

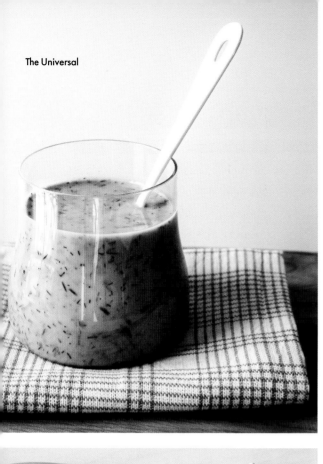

The Universal

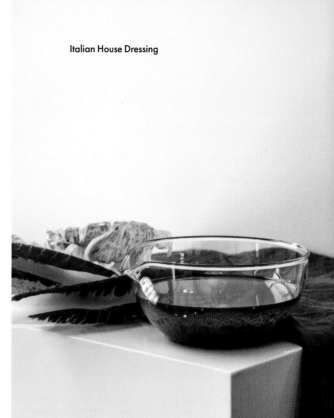

Italian House Dressing

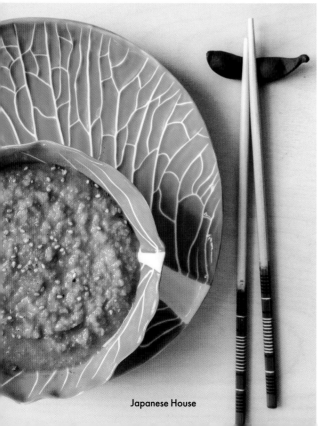

Japanese House

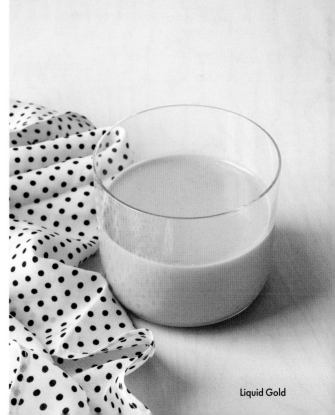

Liquid Gold

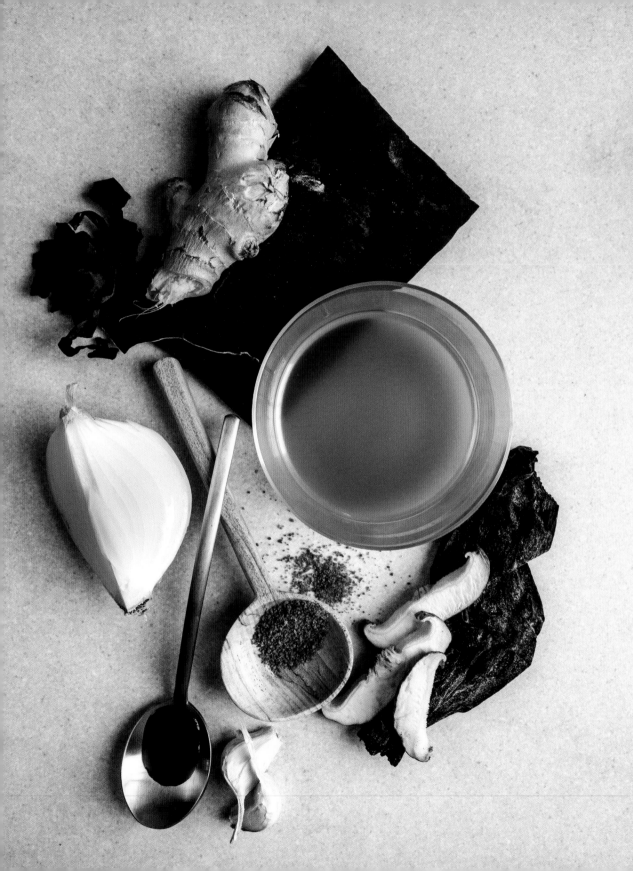

VEGAN FISH SAUCE

This is low-key one of the most important condiments in my pantry. In Southeast Asia, fish sauce is ubiquitous. In Japan, dashi broth (page 159) is as well. You'd be hard pressed to find fully vegan dishes in those parts of the world, save a new wave of plant-based establishments changing the game, because the traditional seafood stock runs centuries deep. The fun thing is, it's really not as hard to replicate as you might think. And you can make a ton and freeze it or keep it in the fridge to add to stocks and stews as you please. Just make sure you keep it in an airtight container because to say the sauce is "fragrant" is a euphemism if there ever was one.

MAKES 2 CUPS (480 ML) SAUCE

INGREDIENTS

1 cup (4 g) dried shiitake or maitake mushrooms, whole

1 sheet kombu

1 tablespoon sea salt

1 tablespoon tamari

3 tablespoons coconut sugar

½ cup (8.5 g) dulse leaves

4 cloves garlic

METHOD

In a saucepan, combine all the ingredients with 2 cups (480 ml) water, bring to a boil, and simmer covered for 30 minutes. Let cool and strain liquid to reserve for sauce. Mushrooms and seaweed can be discarded or blended to add to soups, veggie burgers or stews. Store the sauce in an airtight container in the fridge for up to a week or in the freezer for up to a month.

PEANUT GINGER

I could compare this earthy, salty-sweet dressing to a warm hug. It's comforting but also bright, thanks to the ginger and rice vinegar. It's one of our best sellers at Bonberi Mart. I love it with sturdier greens like kale and cabbage, and it makes an excellent dip for crudités.

MAKES 1¾ CUPS (420 ML) DRESSING

INGREDIENTS

½ cup (120 g) natural creamy or crunchy peanut butter

¼ cup (60 ml) rice vinegar

3 tablespoons maple syrup

¼ cup (60 ml) tamari

2½ teaspoons toasted sesame oil

¾ cup (180 ml) plus 2 tablespoons filtered water

1 teaspoon grated ginger

1 clove garlic, grated

½ teaspoon sea salt

Freshly cracked black pepper

METHOD

In a bowl, whisk the peanut butter, vinegar, syrup, tamari, oil, water, ginger, garlic, and salt until creamy. Season with pepper to taste. Serve over kale salad (page 77) or mung bean noodle salad. You can store the dressing in the fridge in an airtight container for up to 3 days.

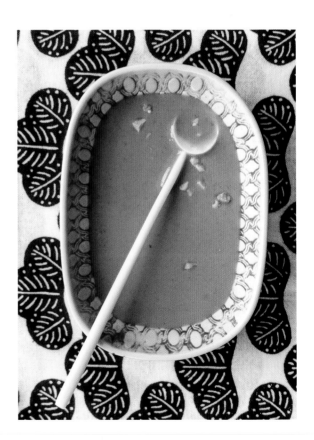

TAHINI GREEN GODDESS

This dressing is summer in a jar. You can certainly make this year-round, and I do! What I love about this so-called recipe is that you can use any variety of fresh herbs that you have on hand and it will be delicious. To make it neutral, you could sub aquafaba mayo for the tahini.

MAKES 1¾ CUPS (420 ML) DRESSING

INGREDIENTS

¼ cup (60 ml) tahini or Aquafaba Mayo (page 223)

1 bunch fresh mint (¾ ounce/5 g)

1 bunch fresh parsley (1 ounce/28 g)

1 bunch fresh dill (1 ounce/28 g)

1 bunch fresh tarragon (⅔ ounce/18 g)

1 bunch fresh basil (¾ ounce/21 g)

2 tablespoons Dijon mustard

½ cup (120 ml) olive oil

2 to 3 cloves garlic

2 tablespoons apple cider vinegar

1 teaspoon lemon zest

1 tablespoon lemon juice

Sea salt

Freshly cracked black pepper

METHOD

In a food processor or blender, blend the tahini, mint, parsley, dill, tarragon, basil, mustard, oil, garlic, vinegar, lemon zest, and lemon juice until creamy. Thin with water, if needed. Season with salt and pepper to taste. Pour over a salad, or serve as a dip for crudités. The dressing will keep in the fridge in an airtight container for up to 3 days.

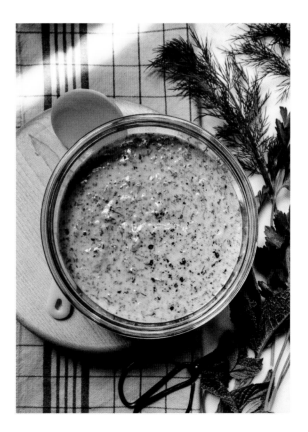

RANCH DRESSING

There is hardly anything more classically American than ranch. I remember being so excited to go to Ruby Tuesday with my dad just because of the salad bar—not because of the salad but because I could pour creamy ranch all over my plate of iceberg, tomato, croutons, and shredded cheddar cheese. (I've come a long way.) At home, we also had that bottle of Hidden Valley ranch and the ominous packets in the cupboard that would magically become an insanely luscious dip just by adding mayo. Well, this recipe is a dead ringer for our childhood favorite, but much better and brighter, thanks to a mix of fresh and dried herbs.

MAKES 2 CUPS (480 ML) DRESSING

INGREDIENTS

1 cup (240 ml) Aquafaba Mayo (page 223) or your favorite store-bought vegan mayo

¼ cup (12 g) fresh dill, finely chopped

½ cup (12 g) fresh chives, finely chopped

¼ cup (12 g) fresh parsley, finely chopped

2 cloves garlic, minced, or ½ teaspoon garlic powder

1 teaspoon onion powder

1 tablespoon apple cider vinegar

½ teaspoon sea salt

Freshly cracked black pepper

METHOD

In a medium bowl, whisk the mayo, dill, chives, parsley, garlic, onion powder, vinegar, and salt with ¼ cup (60 ml) water. (You could also use a blender or food processor.) Season with pepper to taste. The dressing will keep in the fridge in an airtight container for up to 3 days.

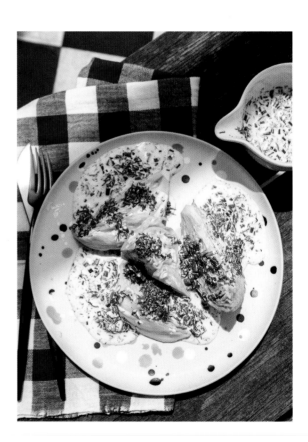

AQUAFABA MAYO

This recipe is a game changer. Leave it to the plant-based scientists (they exist, you know) to figure out that the water left over from canned chickpeas can be whipped into something ethereal, creamy, and heavenly. If you have a couple cans of chickpeas around (and who doesn't?), this mayo counts as an excellent use of food waste. I love to keep a mason jar of it in the fridge to smear on toasts and add to dressings—to anything, really, that needs a good creamy schmear. You'll find that aquafaba mayo is called for quite a bit in this book. Best of all, you never need to buy vegan mayo again. It is creamy, indulgent, and also neutral, so it really goes with any of this book's chapters.

MAKES 2 CUPS (480 ML) MAYO

INGREDIENTS

1 cup aquafaba, from 2 (15-ounce/425-g) cans chickpeas

3 cups (720 ml) avocado oil or cold-pressed olive oil

1 teaspoon sea salt

2 tablespoons apple cider vinegar

2 teaspoons lemon juice

Seasonings (optional)

1 to 2 cloves garlic (to make garlic aioli)

1 teaspoon smoked paprika (to make smoky mayo)

½ teaspoon chipotle chile (to make chipotle mayo)

1 tablespoon wasabi (to make wasabi mayo)

1 jalapeño chile, seeded (to make jalapeño mayo)

1 teaspoon toasted sesame oil (to make Asian mayo)

2 tablespoons ketchup (to make special sauce)

METHOD

In a blender or food processor, blend all the ingredients for up to 5 minutes, until thick. Transfer to an airtight container and store in the fridge for about 6 hours. The mayo will cool and thicken. You can also use an immersion blender for a more whipped, fluffy mayo. Use the optional seasonings to make mayo variations. You can store the mayo in an airtight container in the fridge for up to a week.

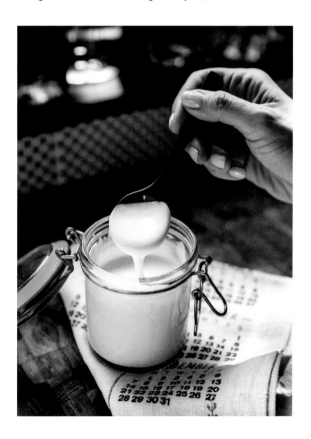

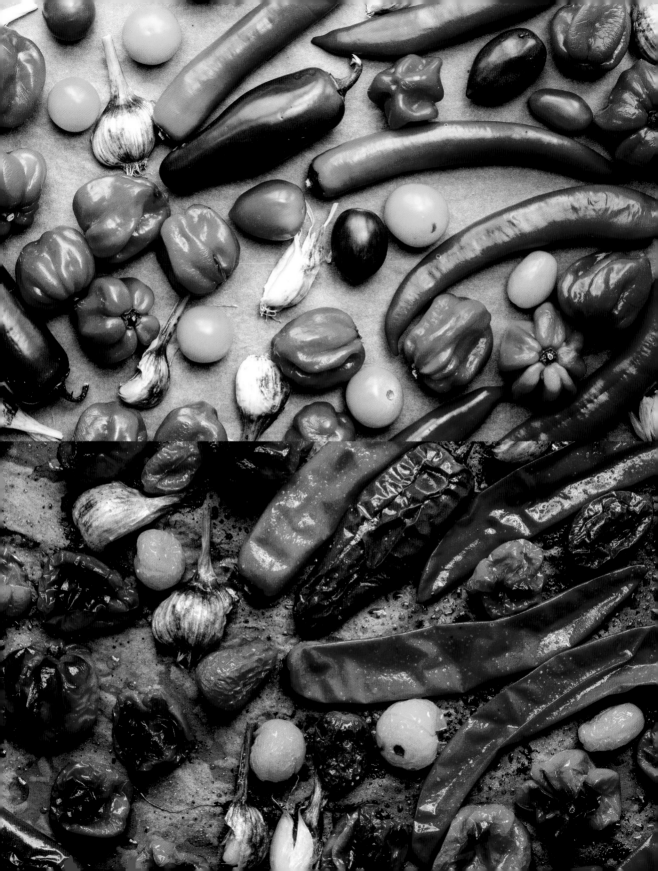

BONBERI HOT SAUCE

I know making your own hot sauce sounds daunting. Why do it when there are endless bottled versions to try? This recipe happened by accident. I am a hot sauce lover, and I love a little heat in almost any dish. One summer, I was grilling hot peppers and I thought, why don't I put them in the blender? I had some cherry tomatoes on hand from the farmers market and threw them in too. The result: Whoa! Tip: When handling this sauce, use gloves. Hot-sauce finger in the eye is not ideal.

MAKES 3 CUPS (720 ML) SAUCE

INGREDIENTS

2 cups (610 g) grape or cherry tomatoes, whole

1½ cups (175 g) hot peppers, such as habanero peppers, cherry peppers, or pimientos

2 tablespoons avocado oil

1 teaspoon sea salt

¼ cup avocado oil

½ medium yellow onion (165 g), peeled and quartered

2 cloves garlic

¼ cup (60 ml) apple cider vinegar

1 teaspoon coconut sugar

METHOD

Preheat the oven to 400°F (205°C). On a parchment-lined baking pan, massage the tomatoes and peppers with the oil and ½ teaspoon of the salt. Roast until browned, 25 to 30 minutes. Let cool.

In a food processor or blender, blend the cooled tomatoes and peppers with the avocado oil, onion, garlic, vinegar, and sugar. Season with the remaining ½ teaspoon of salt, if needed. Blend for 2 to 3 minutes. Refrigerate for 1 hour before serving. The sauce will keep in an airtight container in the fridge for up to a week.

CAVIAR D'AUBERGINES (EGGPLANT CAVIAR)

I studied abroad in Paris when I was twenty-one. My friend Ranya and I lived in an enormous (by college standards) loft-style pied-à-terre in the Marais where we designated an extra bedroom for just our shoes. Yes, we were those girls. This was right when the Marais was becoming THE Marais. There were a couple of galleries and one cool-girl shop on rue Charlot, but for the most part, it was us and the Hasidim, which was fine by me as every Sunday rue des Rosiers would stir with dozens of bustling Jewish *épiceries* peddling Middle Eastern delights. I would hunt and gather mezze, from crispy falafel to tabbouleh to the holy grail—caviar d'aubergines. When I first had this dish, I couldn't get over it. The luscious texture, the salty, smoky goodness, the creamy *tehina*. The umami of it all. All week I looked forward to my Sunday afternoons and that little half pint, which would last me the whole week. It took me years to replicate but I finally brought the flavors back home. This is a bit of a doozy in the kitchen, and a gas stove is recommended (if you don't have one, an oven will do fine). Yes, it's a pain to clean up the charred bits, but whoever is lucky enough to share some crudités and pita with you over this plate will probably not mind being charged with scrubbing the grill later.

To dazzle guests, leave the stem intact and mash the meat of the eggplant, drizzling the sauce ingredients on top and serve with crudités, pita, or crusty bread. For an even creamier version (and the secret to most authentic Israeli versions), add a dollop of vegan mayo.

SERVES 2 TO 3

INGREDIENTS

1 medium to large eggplant (507 g)

¼ cup (60 ml) olive oil

2 tablespoons tahini (or omit to make dish neutral)

¼ cup (12 g) chopped fresh parsley

1 clove garlic, grated

Juice of 1 lemon, or 2 tablespoons lemon juice

½ teaspoon sea salt

Freshly cracked black pepper

Optional

¼ cup (60 ml) Aquafaba Mayo (page 223)

Garnish

1 tablespoon chopped fresh mint leaves

Drizzle of olive oil

For serving

2 Belgian endives, separated into leaves

Crudités

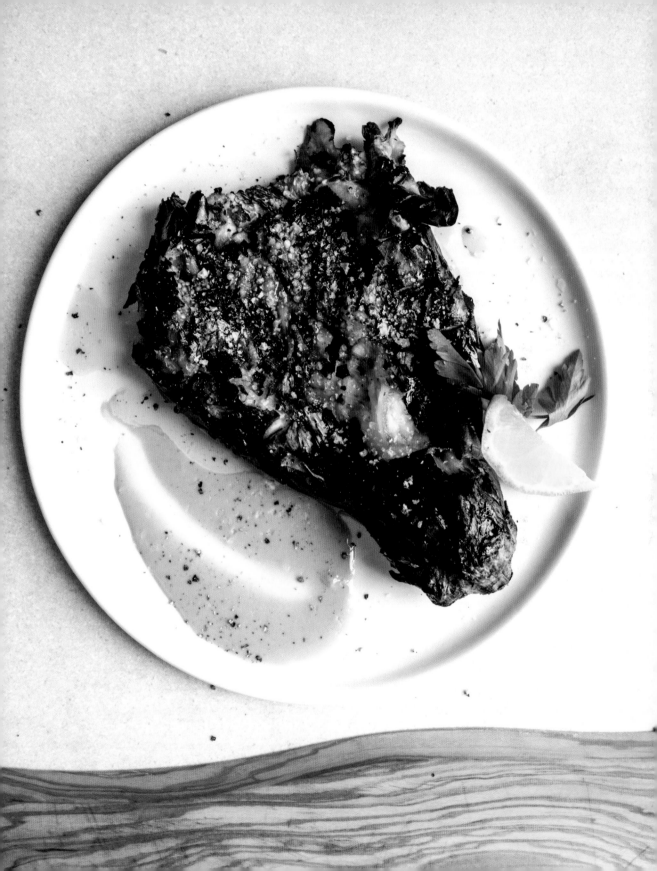

METHOD

To cook the eggplant on a gas stovetop, place it directly on the fire, stem up. Let it sit until the skin begins to char, about 3 minutes. Give it a quarter turn about every 3 minutes, to char each side. Once all the sides are significantly charred, the eggplant should start to shrink. Continue to char and cook the eggplant for about 15 minutes, depending on how strong your flame is. You'll know the eggplant is done when you can easily insert a fork straight through it. If you have a large eggplant and it is not cooking through on the stovetop, bake it in the oven at 425°F (220°C) until tender. With tongs, transfer the eggplant to a shallow bowl and let cool.

If you have a large eggplant and it's not cooking through on the stovetop, char the skin and then transfer to a parchment-lined baking sheet, and bake in the oven. (If you have an electric stovetop, begin at this step.) To do this, preheat the oven to 450°F (230°C). With a fork, poke holes through-out the eggplant, then place it on a baking pan. Put the pan into the oven on the middle shelf, and roast for 30 to 40 minutes, depending on the size of your eggplant. It should begin to shrivel and be easy to pierce with a your fork. For the final 5 minutes, place the eggplant directly under the broiler so that the skin begins to char. Let cool.

Once cool, transfer the eggplant to a cutting board and chop well, making sure you chop through the skin. In a medium bowl, combine the chopped eggplant with the olive oil, tahini (if using), parsley, garlic, lemon juice, and salt and mash with a fork, until well combined. Season with pepper to taste. Add the mayo, if using, for an even creamier caviar. For a smoother texture, transfer the mixture to a food processor or blender.

Transfer the eggplant mixture to a shallow bowl and top with the chopped mint leaves and a drizzle of olive oil. Serve with endive leaves or crudités.

CASHEW RICOTTA

At Bonberi Mart, we use this recipe for nearly everything—as a spread in our club sandwich, as a sub for feta in our Greek salads, and in place of non-vegan ricotta in our Italian Chop at the store. It's so versatile—serve it as a dip too—and you can play with the seasonings and with the texture, depending on how much water you use. Thinned, the ricotta is a great addition to creamy dressings.

It's not mandatory, but the addition of a probiotic will give the ricotta a more tangy, cheese-like flavor. Plus it's great for the gut. If using a probiotic, make sure you stir with a wooden spoon. Metal spoons can interfere with fermenting foods.

MAKES 3 CUPS (720 ML) RICOTTA

INGREDIENTS

3 cups (135 g) raw cashews, soaked overnight or for at least 6 hours

Juice of 1 lemon, or 1½ tablespoons lemon juice

3 cloves garlic

1½ teaspoons nutritional yeast

¼ cup (60 ml) olive oil

Sea salt

2 probiotic capsules

Optional seasonings

Dried oregano

Herbs de Provence

Chipotle powder

Scallions and chives, minced

METHOD

Drain and rinse the cashews. In a food processor or blender, combine the cashews, lemon juice, garlic, yeast, oil, ¼ cup (60 ml) water, and salt to taste. Blend until creamy. Transfer the mixture to an airtight container. Using a wooden spoon, gently stir in the probiotic. Season with the oregano, herbs, chipotle, or scallions, if using. Refrigerate the ricotta overnight before using.

NUT-FREE PESTO

This recipe was born after Nick and I discovered (the hard way) that our son, Jude, had many allergies—including to nuts, seeds, and cheese. I had to get creative and wanted to mimic the creamy texture of pesto without using any of those things. Enter this recipe!

The steamed cauli and zucchini make this sauce "real" pesto's luscious heir apparent, and I steam the garlic to make the sauce more mellow for the little ones. If you're making this for grown-ups, you can absolutely double the garlic and keep it raw for more of a kick. You can also omit the nutritional yeast since this dish is so flavorful on its own.

MAKES 2¾ CUPS (660 ML) SAUCE

INGREDIENTS

1 large zucchini, roughly chopped

1 clove garlic, roughly chopped

2 cups roughly chopped cauliflower florets

2 cups packed baby spinach

Juice of ½ lemon

1 teaspoon sea salt, plus more for seasoning

½ cup packed fresh basil

½ cup (120 ml) olive oil

Freshly cracked black pepper

Optional

2 tablespoons nutritional yeast

METHOD

In a shallow pot or pan fitted with a steamer basket, steam the zucchini, garlic, and cauliflower over 1 inch (2.5 cm) of water. Boil for 10 minutes, or until the vegetables are tender. Remove from the heat and add the spinach; cover and let steam off heat for 3 to 4 minutes more. Uncover to cool. In a blender or food processor, blend the steamed vegetables with the yeast (if using), lemon juice, salt, and basil until creamy. Slowly add in the

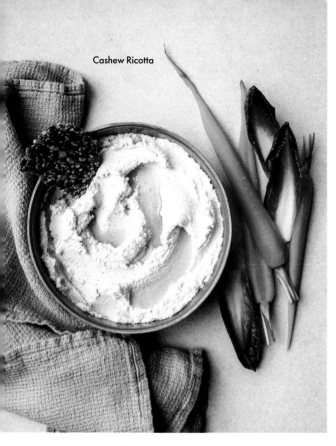
Cashew Ricotta

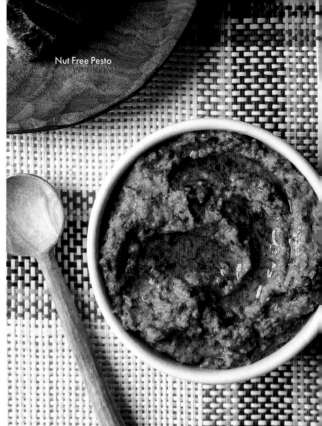
Nut Free Pesto

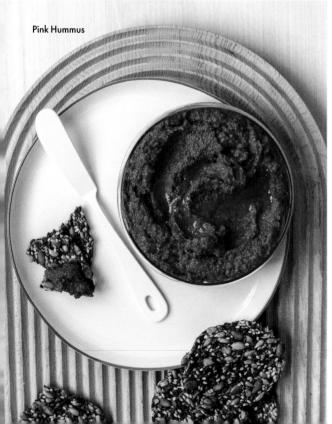
Pink Hummus

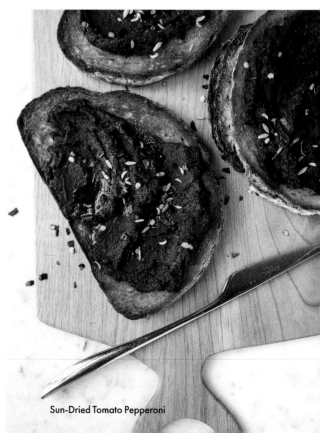
Sun-Dried Tomato Pepperoni

olive oil and continue to blend until you achieve a luscious, creamy texture. Season with sea salt and pepper to taste. The pesto can be frozen for up to 2 weeks for later use

PINK HUMMUS

It stands to reason that every plant-based-cooking blogger has a recipe for pink hummus. It's pretty, it's packed with antioxidants, and, well, it's pretty. My version has a little twist I learned from my friend Ranya's Lebanese mother, Mona. She revealed that the secret to Lebanese hummus is a splash of orange juice. Mind-blowing, right? I went further and added lemon too, with some spices, but the slightly tangy sweetness really vibes well with the naturally sweet beet. Try it for yourself! PS: The ice water trick comes from my friend Danielle's Israeli father, Oded, who taught her that ice water really fluffs up tahini and makes it less dense.

MAKES ROUGHLY 2 CUPS (480 ML) HUMMUS

INGREDIENTS

1 large beet, peeled and chopped into 1-inch (2.5-cm) cubes

2 cloves garlic

1 (15-ounce/425-g) can garbanzo beans, drained and rinsed, or 1½ cups cooked garbanzo beans

2 tablespoons olive oil

1 teaspoon orange zest

Juice of 1 navel orange, or ¼ cup (60 ml) orange juice

1 teaspoon fine sea salt

½ teaspoon sumac

½ teaspoon cumin

¼ cup (60 ml) ice water

2 tablespoons tahini

Juice of ½ lemon

Garnish

1 tablespoon olive oil

1 tablespoon fresh cilantro leaves

1 teaspoon orange zest

Pinch of flaky sea salt

Freshly cracked black pepper

For serving

Crudités (carrots, bell peppers, celery, radish, cucumber)

Tortilla chips

METHOD

In a shallow pot fitted with a steamer basket, bring about 2 inches (5 cm) of water to a boil. Add the beets and steam, covered, on low heat for about 30 minutes, or until tender and easily pierced with a fork. In a food processor, combine the beets with the garlic, beans, oil, orange zest and juice, salt, sumac, cumin, ice water, tahini, and lemon juice until creamy. In a serving bowl, drizzle with the oil and garnish with the cilantro and orange zest. Season with salt and pepper to taste. Serve with crudités or tortilla chips.

SUN-DRIED TOMATO PEPPERONI

Nick, I, and the kids have spent many summers in Ibiza, one of the most magical islands on the planet. I always enjoy discovering new holes-in-the-wall—especially thanks to the island's hippie past, there is plenty of inspiration around every corner. This recipe is based on a sandwich I had in Eivissa, the port town, in a closet of a shop that served a vegan sub-like sandwich. The sign read "vegan pepperoni," which usually means some sort of unidenti-fiable fake meat situation, but when I asked, I was told it was just sun-dried tomatoes. I was baffled. Even more baffled when I ate it. It was one of the best things I had ever tasted. I've dreamed of re-creating it since. The secret is the fennel seeds.

MAKES 1¾ CUPS (420 ML)

INGREDIENTS

1 cup (200 g) packed sun-dried tomatoes, soaked overnight to hydrate, and drained

½ cup (120 ml) olive oil

4 cloves garlic

3 tablespoons fennel seeds

½ teaspoon ground mustard powder

½ teaspoon sea salt

1 teaspoon red chili flakes

¼ cup (12 g) fresh parsley, chopped

Freshly cracked black pepper

METHOD

In a food processor, combine the tomatoes, oil, garlic, fennel seeds, mustard powder, salt, chili flakes, parsley, and ¼ cup (120 ml) or more water, as needed. Pulse until a tapenade-like paste forms. Season with pepper to taste. Serve the pepperoni as a dip, on crackers, or in a sandwich. It can keep in the fridge for up to 3 days.

ISRAELI-STYLE AVOCADO HUMMUS

I gave this recipe its name because while on vacation in Israel in my early twenties, I learned that Israelis overcook their chickpeas in order to create this fluffy, cloud-like version (which also saves the time needed to peel off the skin of every garbanzo bean, which is a cheerless task.) The avocados were originally just impro-vised—I had a few about to go bad so I threw them in there—but the result was a creamy plate of goodness that I wanted to re-create again and again. Tip: Add a little tahini drizzle for extra presentation points. For combining, it's ideal with crudités.

SERVES 4

INGREDIENTS

For the hummus

2 teaspoons baking soda

½ teaspoon fine sea salt (for the water)

1 (15-ounce/425-g) can chickpeas, drained and rinsed, or 1½ cups cooked chickpeas

¼ cup (60 ml) olive oil

Juice of 1 lemon, or 2 tablespoons lemon juice

2 tablespoons tahini

2 avocados

2 cloves garlic

Sea salt

Freshly cracked black pepper

¼ cup (60 ml) ice water

For the tahini topping

3 tablespoons tahini

¼ cup (60 ml) ice water

1 ice cube

1 clove garlic, grated

Sea salt

Freshly cracked black pepper

Garnish

Fresh Parsley

Fresh Mint

Smoked paprika

Olive oil

Flaky Salt

Black Pepper

METHOD

Make the hummus: In a medium pot, add the baking soda and salt to 4 to 6 cups (960 ml to 1.4 L) water and bring to a boil. Add the chickpeas and keep on a low rolling boil for 20 minutes, being careful not to let the water boil over. Drain the chickpeas and let cool slightly. Once the chickpeas have cooled, but are still warm, transfer them to a food processor and add the oil, lemon juice, tahini, avocados, garlic, and salt and pepper to taste. While blending, slowly add the ice water. Blend to a thick, velvety consistency, and set aside.

Make the tahini topping: In a medium bowl, combine the tahini, ice water, ice cube, garlic, and salt and pepper to taste. Whisk vigorously, with the ice cube in the bowl, until creamy and fluffy. You want the topping to have a light, airy consistency. If it is too dense, you can add more ice water.

To serve, transfer the hummus to a shallow serving bowl with a spatula and spoon the tahini mixture on top. Add your garnish and serve with toast, pita, chips, and crudités.

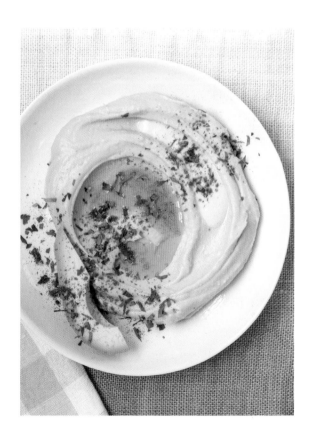

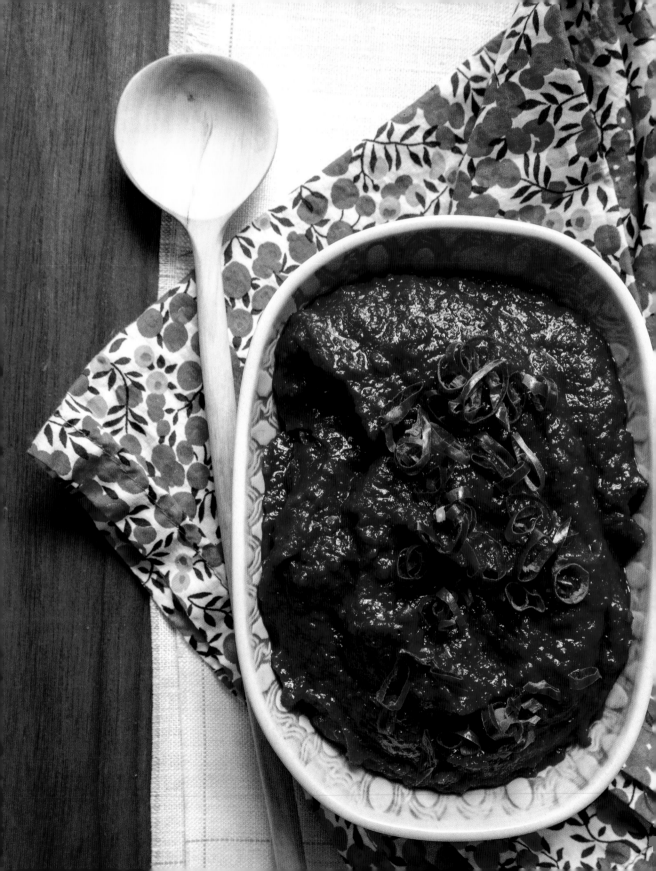

BEET GOCHUJANG

This is one of my favorite condiments used in Korean cooking. It lends luscious umami, spicy, salty-sweet goodness to anything it touches. You can add it to noodles, rice dishes, stews, roasted cauliflower, and even wraps or sandwiches. It's not easy to source store-bought versions that don't contain corn syrup, dyes, or other additives, and I was shocked at how easy it is to replicate at home without compromising on flavor. The addition of steamed chopped beets brings a vibrant hot pink hue, which I find a bit unexpected and fun.

MAKES 1½ CUPS (360 ML) GOCHUJANG

INGREDIENTS

¼ cup (38 g) steamed chopped beets

2-inch (5-cm) knob ginger, peeled and grated, or 1 teaspoon grated ginger

1 clove garlic

¼ cup (60 ml) maple syrup

½ teaspoon cayenne pepper, or 1 teaspoon gochugaru (Korean red pepper flakes)

2 teaspoons toasted sesame oil

½ cup (120 ml) red or white miso paste

2 tablespoons tamari

¼ cup (60 ml) rice vinegar

2 scallions, chopped

Optional

½ teaspoon sea salt

METHOD

In a blender, combine the beets, ginger, garlic, syrup, cayenne, oil, miso paste, tamari, and vinegar. Slowly add ½ cup (60 ml) water and blend until creamy. Add the salt, if using. Transfer the paste to a small bowl and, using a spoon or spatula, gently add the scallions. The gochujang will keep in the fridge in an airtight container for up to a week.

CHOPPED LIVER

This recipe is an ode to my dad. When I was younger, on the Jewish High Holidays my dad and I would sneak snacks of chopped liver and crackers, waiting for dinner to begin. We would snack and get full and then get scolded . . . but he'd throw a sly smirk my way, and it felt good. I've put a veggie spin on the classic chopped liver, featuring powerhouse plant ingredients like brown lentils and walnuts, and the dupe is kind of extraordinary.

MAKES 3 CUPS

INGREDIENTS

6 tablespoons (90 ml) avocado oil

1 large yellow or white onion, chopped, or 2 cups (420 g) chopped onion

2 cloves garlic, minced

1 tablespoon tamari

2 cups (150 g) brown lentils, cooked

1 cup (105 g) raw walnuts

1 teaspoon sea salt

1 teaspoon ground black pepper

Garnish

Freshly chopped parsley

METHOD

In a large saucepan, heat 2 tablespoons (30 ml) of the oil. Add the onion, garlic, and tamari and sauté on medium-high heat for 5 to 7 minutes, until cooked down. Let cool. Transfer the onion mixture to a food processor or blender and add the lentils, walnuts, the remaining 4 tablespoons (60 ml) of the oil, the salt, and pepper. Blend until creamy. Serve as a dip with crudites or use as a "pate" spread on a banh mi (see page 199).

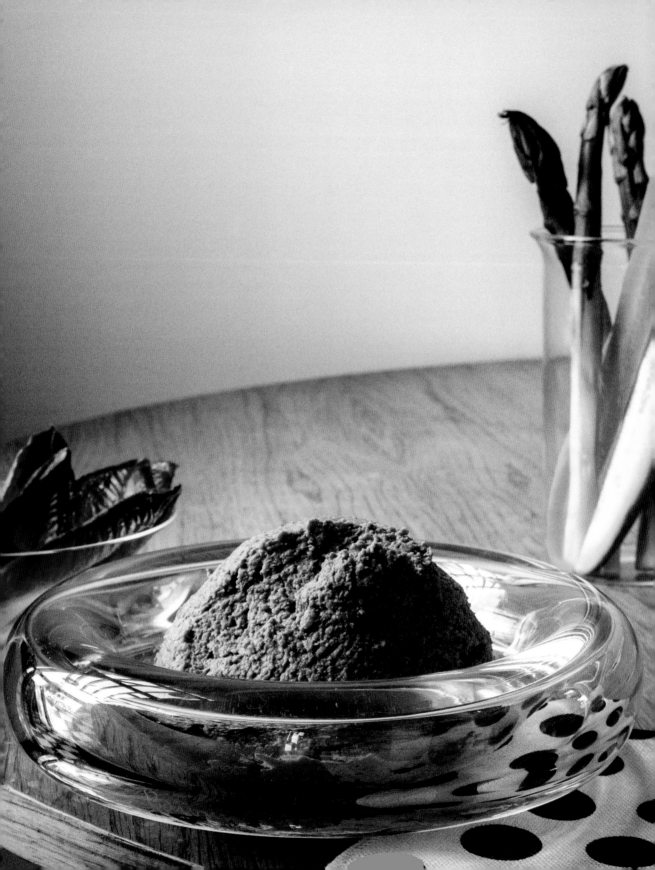

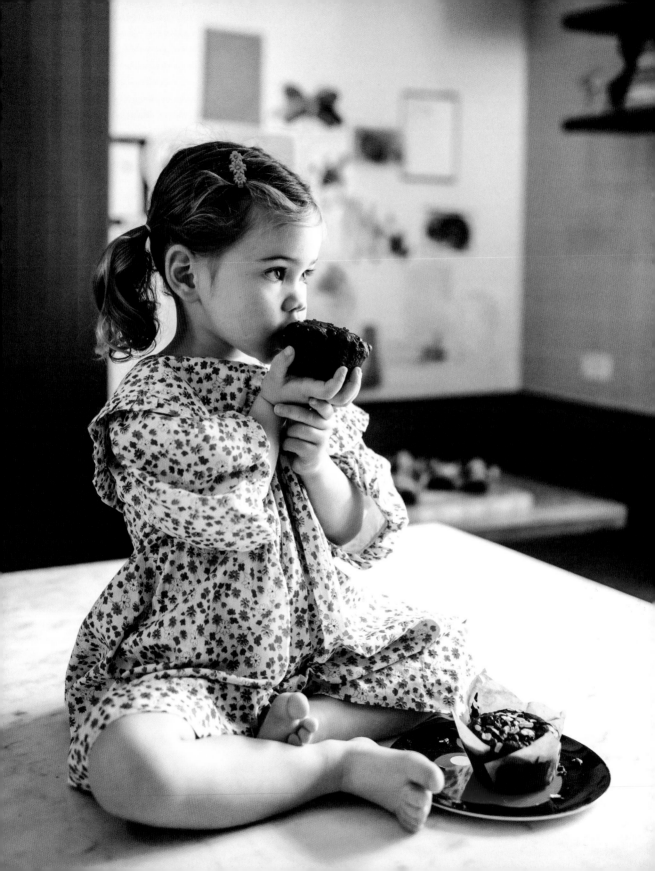

SWEETS

BONBERI COCONUT GRANOLA

I have always loved granola but have also always felt run-down after having it, as if there was a pit in my stomach, and it's no wonder why. Though deemed "health food," granola is usually a food-combining nightmare, mixing fruit, nuts, and oats—literally creating a pit in your stomach. This recipe is a spin on one of my favorite granolas and is properly food-combined while also being grain- and nut-free. It's the perfect combination of salty and sweet, which makes it entirely appropriate for a topping over coconut yogurt, dessert or even a cereal-for-dinner meal with some plant-based milk. Yum.

SERVES 6 TO 8

INGREDIENTS

3 cups (270 g) unsweetened coconut flakes (Let's Do Organic brand is great.)

¼ cup (50 g) chia seeds

¼ cup (40 g) hemp seeds

½ teaspoon sea salt

½ teaspoon ground cinnamon

⅛ teaspoon ground cardamom

1 teaspoon grated fresh ginger

1 tablespoon orange zest

¼ cup (60 ml) orange juice

½ cup (120 ml) maple syrup

2 tablespoons coconut oil, melted

METHOD

Preheat the oven to 375°F (190°C). If your oven runs hot, set it to 350°F (175°C).

In a large bowl, combine dry ingredients: coconut, seeds, salt, and spices and set aside. In a medium mixing bowl, combine the grated ginger, orange zest, orange juice, syrup, and coconut oil and whisk until well emulsified. Pour over dry ingredients in large bowl and massage well with your hands until fully coated.

Line a 18 by 13-inch (46 by 33-cm) baking sheet with parchment paper and evenly spread the granola mixture flat onto the pan. Bake until lightly browned, about 15 minutes. Using a wooden spoon or spatula, toss gently to bring up white/uncooked granola and bake for 5 to 10 minutes more. You want most of the granola to be lightly browned. Let cool for 20 to 30 minutes to allow it to crisp up. The granola will keep in an airtight container unrefrigerated for about 1 week.

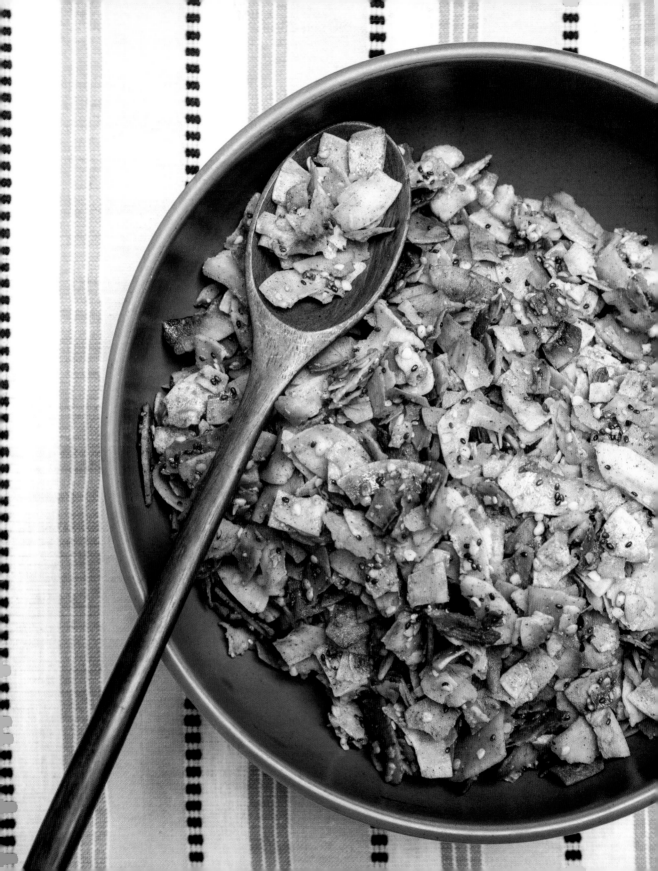

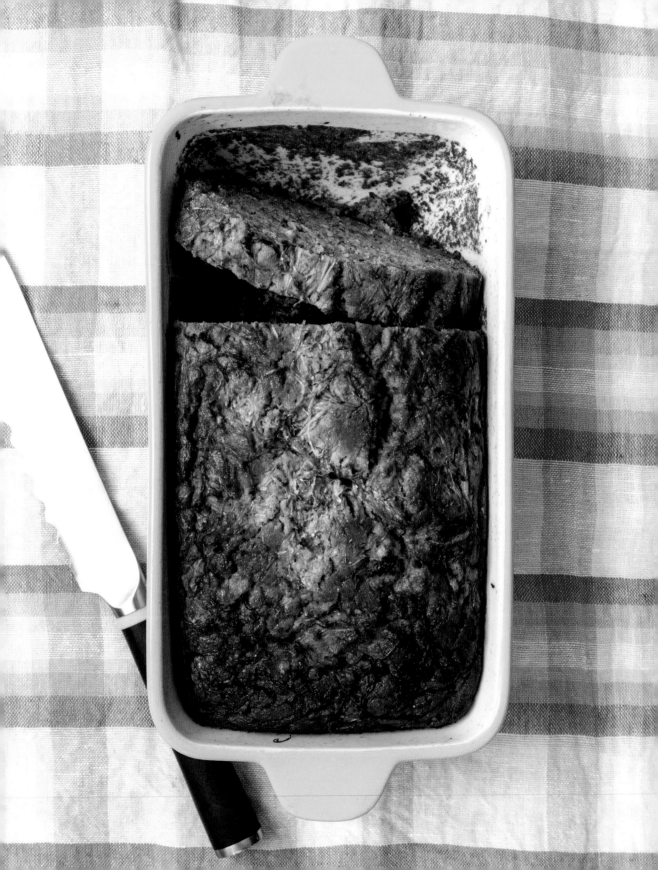

ZUCCHINI BREAD

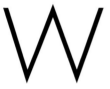hat I love about this loaf is it's actually properly food-combined. Bananas are starchier than typical fruits, so they combine well with starch. It's my favorite sweet treat and the first that I gave to both my kids, while also serving them a dose of veggies.

SERVES 6 TO 8

INGREDIENTS

¼ cup (60 ml) coconut oil, melted, plus more for the pan

3 tablespoons ground flax seeds

¼ cup (60 ml) warm water

1 cup (240 ml) maple syrup

1 teaspoon vanilla extract

2 very ripe bananas, mashed

2 zucchini, grated

1½ cups (10½ ounces/295 g) white rice flour

1½ cups (8 ounces/225 g) garbanzo bean flour

½ teaspoon baking powder

¼ teaspoon baking soda

1 teaspoon ground cinnamon

1 teaspoon ground nutmeg

½ teaspoon salt

METHOD

Preheat the oven to 350°F (175°C). Grease a loaf pan with coconut oil.

Combine the flax seeds and warm water. Wait until it forms the consistency of an egg. In a large bowl, combine the flax egg, syrup, ¼ cup oil, and vanilla. Beat well. Stir in the mashed bananas and grated zucchini.

In a separate bowl, whisk the flours, baking powder, baking soda, cinnamon, nutmeg, and salt. Add the dry mixture to the wet and stir just until the dry ingredients are moistened and everything is incorporated evenly. Pour the batter into the prepared pan.

Bake for 50 minutes, or until a knife inserted in the center of the loaf comes out clean. Let cool before slicing. Enjoy!

JUDE'S FRENCH TOAST

This recipe was born from my son Jude's allergies, which prevented him from having eggs and lots of other breakfast foods. It's so simple and makes the most decadent French toast. In fact, we make it a few times a week. This is an example of when a nontoxic nonstick pan would do well.

SERVES 2

INGREDIENTS

2 ripe bananas

½ teaspoon ground cinnamon

1 cup (240 ml) almond milk or oat milk

1 tablespoon avocado oil, grass-fed butter, ghee, or coconut oil for frying

4 slices millet bread, thawed

Optional toppings

½ teaspoon ground cinnamon

Handful of blueberries or raspberries

Sliced banana

1 tablespoon raw almond butter

Maple syrup

METHOD

In a blender or food processor, blend the bananas, cinnamon, and milk. Pour into a large shallow bowl.

Heat up a skillet. Add butter or oil to the skillet to melt on medium-high heat. Dip the slices of bread in the banana mixture and let them soak up liquid on both sides. Add the drenched bread to the skillet and cook until browned on both sides, about 1 minute each.

Garnish with optional toppings, in whatever combination you like. Add maple syrup and enjoy!

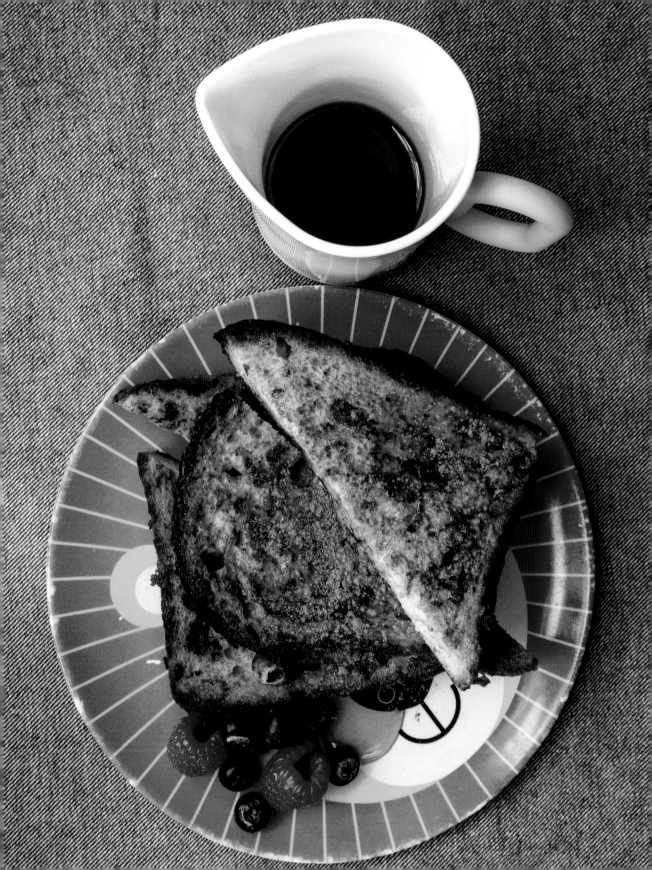

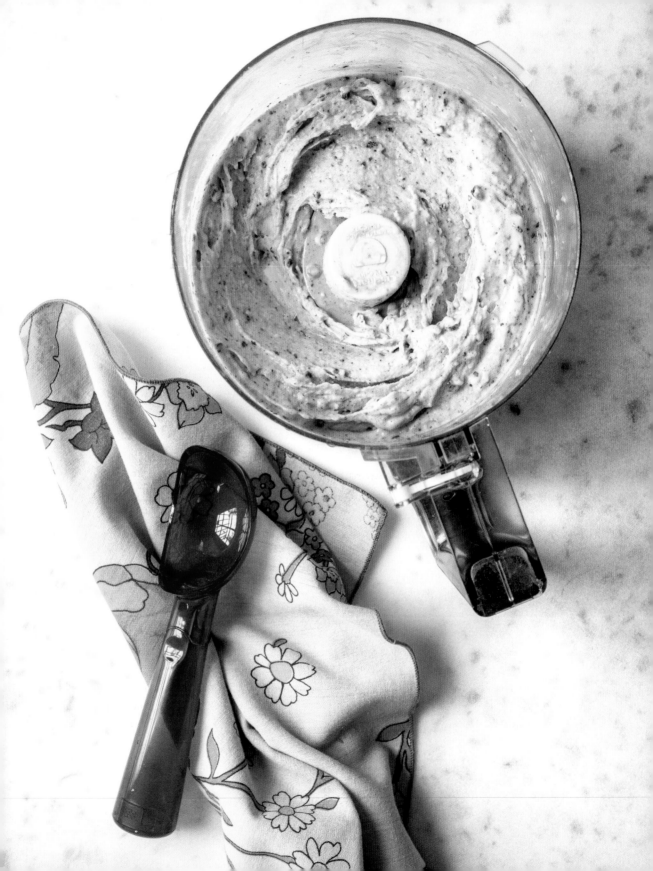

CHUNKY MONKEY FROYO

Once you've had this banana "froyo," you won't want the original again. These days there are many great nondairy alternatives to ice cream, but they're usually quite heavy, made with coconut or cashew. I, for one, feel worse after I have them. Since banana is starchier than most fruit, this is a good entry-level dessert after a starch or raw meal. You can even have it for breakfast, subbing more fruit for the chocolate. Yes, the peanut butter and nuts are a slight food combining bend, but it's ice cream, so it's worth it.

MAKES 1 CUP

INGREDIENTS

2 extra-ripe bananas (245 g)

2 tablespoons raw almonds

2 tablespoons peanut butter

2 tablespoons dark chocolate chips

Dash of sea salt

METHOD

Twelve hours or the night before, peel and slice the bananas. Store in the freezer.

When you're ready to prepare the froyo, in a food processor or high-quality blender, combine the bananas, almonds, peanut butter, chocolate chips, and sea salt. Feel free to add more toppings. I love cinnamon and shredded raw coconut! Blend until creamy. Best served immediately.

JUICE PULP MUFFINS

A few years ago, I volunteered to bring muffins for my son Jude's preschool bake sale. I'm always looking to incorporate more vegetables into my kids' diet, and this is the perfect sneaky way to do it. You can grate zucchini right in or, for a more sustainable version, save the pulp of your daily green juice to mix in for a nutrient-packed treat. We've since made these a staple at Bonberi Mart and sell out every morning and I can thank our head cook Marlen Fernandez for taking the recipe to the next level. And since most school are nut-free, these are also mostly allergen friendly, if you opt for rice or oat milk.

MAKES 6 LARGE MUFFINS

INGREDIENTS

1 cup (240ml) oat milk or rice milk

½ cup olive oil

½ cup maple syrup

1 teaspoon vanilla extract

¼ cup cold brew

½ cup coconut sugar

2½ cups gluten-free all purpose flour

¼ cup unsweetened cocoa powder

2 tablespoons baking powder

1 tablespoon baking soda

¼ teaspoon salt

½ cup juice pulp or grated zucchini

½ cup dark chocolate chips

For Toping

1 teaspoon coconut sugar

1 teaspoon rolled oats

1 tablespoon dark chocolate chips

METHOD

Preheat oven to 375. In a large bowl, whisk the milk, oil, syrup, vanilla, cold brew and combine well. In a separate bowl, combine the sugar, flour, cocoa powder, baking powder, baking soda, and salt. Slowly add the dry ingredients to the wet ingredients and combine well with a spatula. Fold in juice pulp or drain the grated zucchini, if using, removing excess liquid, and fold into the batter. Fold in chocolate chips.

Place cupcake liners in a cupcake tin and scoop batter into each liner, filling it to the top. Sprinkle sugar, oats and chocolate chips evenly over muffins.

Bake for 35 minutes, or until a toothpick inserted in the middle comes out clean. Let cool and enjoy!

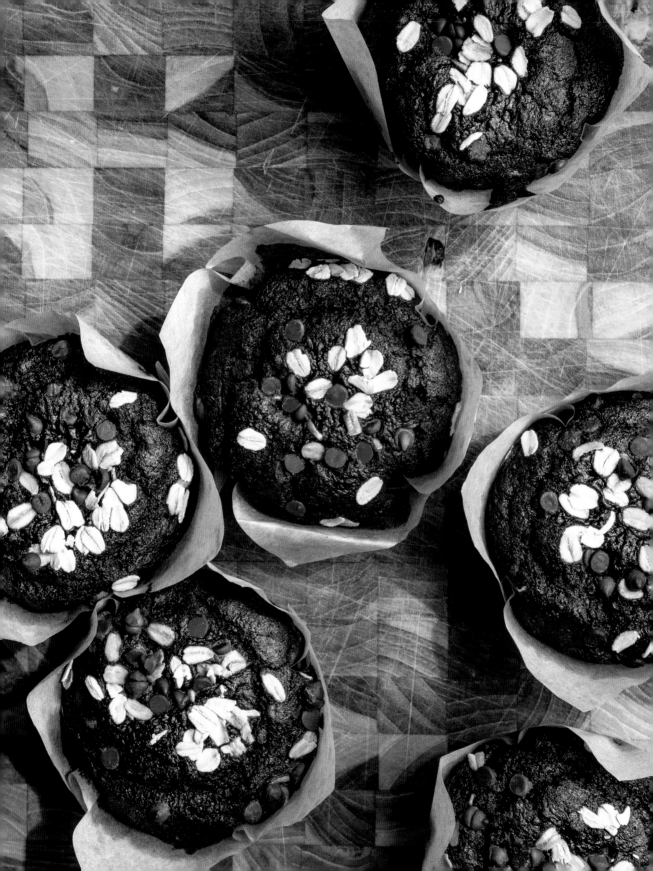

CHOCOLATE AVOCADO MOUSSE

Although there aren't many sweets in this book, I do love some dark rich chocolate, and this reminds me of the kind of mousse that I used to order at restaurants as a kid and that came in a fancy glass. It's ideal after a starchy meal. The espresso is not required but does lend a richness to the pudding.

MAKES 1¾ CUPS MOUSSE

INGREDIENTS

2 avocados, pitted

2 heaping tablespoons cacao powder

¼ cup (60 ml) maple syrup

1 tablespoon espresso, or 2 tablespoons cold brew (optional)

½ teaspoon ground cinnamon

1 teaspoon vanilla extract

Dash of salt

Optional

1 tablespoon peanut butter

METHOD

In a blender or food processor, blend the avocados, cacao powder, syrup, ¼ cup (60 ml) water, espresso, peanut butter (if using), cinnamon, vanilla, and salt. Enjoy immediately or keep in the fridge in an airtight container for up to 3 days.

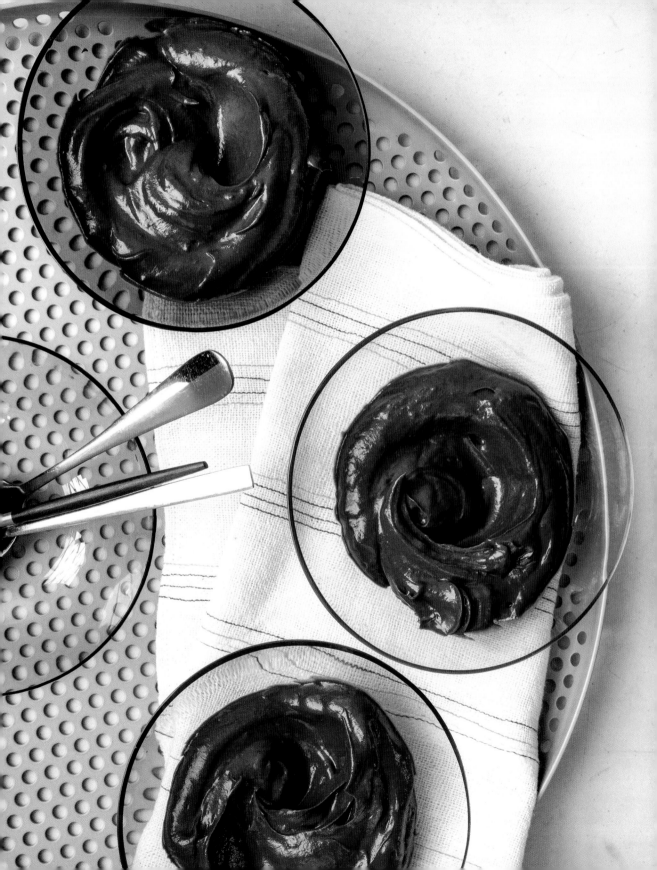

EXTRA CREDIT: ALL ABOUT SELF-CARE

She was becoming herself and daily casting aside that fictitious self which we assume like a garment with which to appear before the world.

—KATE CHOPIN, *The Awakening*

MY LIFE TOOK A NOTABLE TURN FOR THE BETTER the moment I took my self-care as seriously as I took my work. I made feeling good the priority. I'm not saying we all should check out and abandon our responsibilities to get massages and facials 24/7. This is not the self-care I speak of. The self-care I speak of is doing the things that feel good in the moment.

Other radical acts of self-care? Slowing down when our bodies give us signals that we are going too fast. Taking a moment to breathe in the morning. Deciding to cook your own meals for a few days a week instead of ordering takeout. Alone time. These small acts of kindness to ourselves are the ultimate acts of self-care.

Think of yourself as that little kid again. Many of us grew up with someone looking after us. Feeding us when we were hungry, drawing us a warm bath after we got caught in the rain, and putting us to bed when we were overtired. In adulthood, we must become our own parents, our own caretakers looking out for ourselves. When we grow up, we are expected to take the hits, tough it up, walk it off. We are made to believe we must white-knuckle our way through life and success is only worth it if it took a lot of blood, sweat, and tears. But as I've achieved more success in my life and career, I've come to realize that could not be further from the truth. The more I care for myself, the more able and grounded I am to conquer what lies before me.

Self-care can mean so many things. It can mean saying no. It can mean watching your favorite show. It can mean going to your favorite spa or taking a bath. There is no wrong self-care so long as it does not slow or hinder our healing process.

Exfoliation

This might come from my childhood memories of my Korean mother vigorously scrubbing my skin with a sandpaper-like cloth to remove dead skin, but exfoliation, to me, is the ultimate beauty technique, and costs almost nothing. I like to think of food combining and juicing as inner exfoliation, helping scrub our insides of accumulated waste. I feel the same way about the skin! Of course, the skin is one of the largest organs of the body, so it's important for me to allow my skin to breathe. I do this by using natural beaded cleansers, serums that contain vitamin C and fruit acids to help generate skin and cellular renewal, and actual exfoliators like Korean washcloths.

Dry brushing—using a natural bristle brush to slough dead skin—is also an excellent way to remove dead skin, increase lymphatic flow, and boost circulation. The best way to dry brush? I like to do it to increase circulation first thing in the morning—it's better than an espresso shot! Remember not to use any oils or creams that can clog the pores, as the goal is ultimately to open the pores in your skin so they can breathe. Remember to always brush upward from your feet toward the heart, and down the arms, toward the heart, and clockwise in circular motions on your stomach center. This is one of my essential daily self-care practices. Using a dry natural bristle brush over the body on a regular basis will improve circulation in the skin and cells by providing lymphatic drainage. The bristles also remove dead layers of skin, which helps detoxification. The benefits? Smoother skin, better circulation, and reduction of cellulite.

Exercise

For me, daily movement is absolutely essential for achieving body harmony. But I will also say that if you don't love your workout, it will do anything but lend balance. I remember the years of toiling on a StairMaster or treadmill. Luckily, I found a workout I absolutely love that incorporates dancing elements that make me feel free and make my soul sing. I look forward to doing it every day. I also love yoga, particularly hot yoga, where you leave everything on the mat. I encourage you to experiment with different frameworks to find the right one for you.

When I am on vacation, particularly at the beach, I love to jog and explore any nearby city. Movement is also an opportunity to become intuitive.

Colonic Hydrotherapy

I have for years coupled colonic treatments with an alkaline lifestyle, and I truly believe in their healing efficacy. For me, the most effective method of colonics is the Gravity Method, which uses a gentle flow of water to remove excess waste. I assure those wary of colonics: It simply uses the power of gravity. (A tank of water suspended above the body enters the body, and elimination exits through a tube with the help of gravity and water.) It can actually be quite relaxing, and the pay-off once you get off the table is clear. After a successful colonic session, you can feel clear-headed, energized, and certainly lighter.

Of course, if this is outside your comfort zone, at-home enemas are an option for which you can purchase kits at your local drug store. But no matter how you do it, elimination is key.

Far Infrared Saunas

Unlike Finnish saunas, which use heated coals to heat the air, far infrared saunas use light to penetrate human tissue—actually raising the body's core temperature. The result? A deeper detox that can aid in weight loss and inflammation, sleep, and stress reduction, and that can even support the immune system. Remember, the key to Body Harmony is elimination, and elimination includes sweat. When we sweat, we are able to release toxins through our skin.

Korean Body Scrubs

I grew up going to Korean bathhouses with my mom. The art of public bathing is an honored tradition in many Asian cultures, and for good reason. The saunas bring forth a deep detoxifying sweat, and alternating between hot and cold plunges acts as intense lymphatic draining, expanding and contracting the cells for optimal detoxification. At Korean spas, they also offer body scrubs, which are an integral part of my self-care and detoxifying lifestyle. The process consists of intensely scrubbing the skin with an exfoliating loofah until shreds of dead skin are removed. Our skin is the biggest organ of our body, so you can imagine how many toxins from creams, sweat, dirt, and environmental pollution can accumulate. And the proof is in the pudding. After one treatment you feel your skin breathe like it never has before. Check whether there are any Korean or Russian spas near you. If not, you can do your own home treatment—dry brushing followed by hot and freezing-cold intervals in the shower—for a similar result.

Seaweed and Clay Wraps

Body wraps definitely call to mind traditional spas of the 1980s with women decked out in curlers, cucumber rounds on top of their closed eyes. But seaweed wraps are wonderfully effective at pulling out impurities from the skin and infusing the body with mineral-rich nutrients. To do this at home, purchase a jar of French or bentonite clay, mix it with a little water and cover your skin, then sit in your bathtub (this can get messy!) for about thirty minutes. Afterward your skin will be baby soft and you'll feel your energy skyrocket.

Salt Baths

I love Epsom salt baths during the winter. They can be incredibly detoxifying and soothing thanks to the natural magnesium. (Magnesium also promotes elimination.) Start off small as the detoxifying effect can make you light-headed.

Coffee Scrubs

I love this at-home treatment because it's so easy and so effective. The salt will draw out any water retention, the caffeine stimulates and tightens the body, and the coconut oil leaves your skin feeling silky smooth. Just combine 1 cup ground coffee beans, 1 cup coconut oil, and ½ cup Epsom salts in a large bowl and mix well until it forms a delicious-smelling paste. In the bathtub or shower, scoop up handfuls of the paste and rub it all over your body, focusing on areas that are retaining water, like your belly, bum, thighs, and upper arms. Rub vigorously in circular motions on your body to exfoliate. Sit in the tub for five or ten minutes and then rinse off.

Lymphatic Massage / Shiatsu Massage

I grew up with bodywork as an important part of life. My mother would take us to Chinese doctors who would press pressure points in our hands to get rid of headaches. (I remember crying out in defiance at the time, but now I'm grateful.) In the modern world, whether due to stress, sitting at a desk for hours at a time, or just everyday life, our bodies tend to stagnate. It is important to help the energy and blood flow easily and without blockage. Massage is an excellent way to promote circulation. I don't mean the fancy types of massage where they slather on expensive oils. I mean deep tissue massage, often called shiatsu, sports massage, or tui na. I actually ask that the therapist not use any oils since the whole point is to open the body, not clog it with synthetic creams. If you have budget constraints or can't get yourself to a spa, a way to get this deep massage effect at home is to invest in a firm foam roller.

One of my favorite things about this lifestyle is how seamlessly you can incorporate it into the outside world and fully immerse yourself in living your life. This is what has kept me consistent for years on end: being able to participate fully in the joys of life.

ACKNOWLEDGMENTS

I want to thank all the people who have helped in the creation of this book, which spans long before I even began writing the book.

To my teachers: Gabby, Gil, Natalia, Jamie. Thank you for opening my eyes to a new way of living and thriving. I will always be your student and humbled by your commitment to true health and living life in the truest form.

To my book team: Sasha, Jason, Randi, Jessica Jane, Marlen, and Mariah. Thank you for devoting an (intense) week of your lives to create the beauty that is this book. I'll always remember our eight days in Brooklyn! A special thank you to my brother Scott for letting me use his kitchen to test recipes and Sam and Mitch for opening their beautiful home to us with such generosity and grace. And a big thank-you to Holly, my very first book editor, for schooling me on how the proverbial (vegan) sausage is made. Thank you to Danielle Duboise for believing this book should even exist.

To my family: Nick, Jude, Sea for bearing with me during these long months whether it was recipe testing, editing, shooting, thank you for being the force behind all of this and truly the only reason I keep striving for more. Thank you to my mom and brothers for always believing in me and my late-bloomer-ness, and to my dad, who had his hand on my shoulder every step of the way.

Lastly, I have so much humble gratitude to the Bonberi community that has grown over the years on social media and beyond. You guys are the reason this book exists and inspire me every day to create and share more. Each page in this book is my thank you to each and every one of you for believing and supporting Bonberi over the years. THANK YOU!

SOURCES AND FURTHER READING

The Enzyme Factor, by Hiromi Shinya, MD
Detox for Women, by Natalia Rose
The Miracle of Mindfulness, by Thich Nhat Hanh
Peace Is Every Step, by Thich Nhat Hanh
A Return To Love, by Marianne Williamson
A Course In Miracles, by the Foundation for Inner Peace
The Power of Now, by Eckhart Tolle
You Can Heal Your Life, by Louise Hay
Become Younger, by Norman W. Walker, MD
The Mucusless Diet, by Arnold Ehret

Editor: Holly Dolce
Designer: Heesang Lee
Managing Editor: Mike Richards
Production Manager: Larry Pekarek

Library of Congress Control Number: 2021946808

ISBN: 978-1-4197-5649-8
eISBN: 978-1-64700-688-4

Printed and bound in the United States
10 9 8 7 6 5 4 3 2 1

Abrams books are available at special discounts when purchased in quantity for
premiums and promotions as well as fundraising or educational use. Special editions can
also be created to specification. For details, contact specialsales@abramsbooks.com or
the address below.

Abrams® is a registered trademark of Harry N. Abrams, Inc.

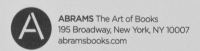

ABRAMS The Art of Books
195 Broadway, New York, NY 10007
abramsbooks.com